Children, teenagers and health
THE KEY DATA

Children, teenagers and health
THE KEY DATA

Caroline Woodroffe, Myer Glickman,
Maggie Barker and Chris Power

Research Consultant: Madeleine Simms

Open University Press
Buckingham · Philadelphia

Open University Press
Celtic Court
22 Ballmoor
Buckingham
MK18 1XW

and

1900 Frost Road, Suite 101
Bristol, PA 19007, USA

First Published 1993
Reprinted 1995

A catalogue record of this book is available from the British Library

ISBN 0 335 19125 8 (pb)

Library of Congress Cataloging-in-Publication Data
Children, teenagers and health: the key data/by Caroline Woodroffe [*et al.*].
    p.   cm.
  Includes bibliographical references and index.
  ISBN 0-335-19125-8
  1. Children – Health and hygiene – Great Britain – Statistics.
2. Teenagers – Health and hygiene – Great Britain – Statistics.
I. Woodroffe, Caroline, 1938–.
RJ103.G7C5   1993
362.1′9892′000941021 – dc20   93-16795   CIP

Typeset by Vision Typesetting, Manchester
Printed in Great Britain by St Edmundsbury Press Ltd,
Bury St Edmunds, Suffolk

Contents

Foreword

It is from studies of children that we have learnt most about the importance of non-medical influences on health and development. Parental education, culture and occupation, socio-economic conditions, housing and prevailing political values all play major parts in determining the short- and long-term physical, mental and psychological development of these most vulnerable members of society.

However, in spite of the massive amount of statistical data available in the UK on the health of children and their families, little has been done to pull together in one place relevant data from the variety of sources that produce it, often stemming from different Government and private agencies. This has been the aim of this publication, which includes data from such Government Departments as Health, Social Security, Transport and Environment, as well as from numerous research sources such as the national birth cohorts and morbidity surveys. Even with the net cast as widely as it has been, there are certainly areas of interest not covered, but this well-illustrated account demonstrates beyond question the breadth of the interests which reflect on the health of children.

The message to policy-makers is clear. There is scarcely a field in which the interest of children does not need to be considered, taking into account possible effects both on their current health and on the health of the adults that they will become. Equally, these facts need to be known to those responsible for all levels of relevant educational programmes. This book should become an essential reference source for these and all others concerned with the health of children.

Professor Eva Alberman

Acknowledgements

We have benefited from the guidance of the Wolfson Child Health Monitoring Unit Advisory Committee: Eva Alberman (Chair), Jean Chapple, Ian Lister Cheese (on scientific matters), Catherine Peckham.

Many colleagues in the Institute of Child Health have contributed to this book: Elizabeth Anionwu, Helen Bedford, Clare Davison, Carol Dezateux, Ruth Gilbert, Philip Graham, Gill Jones, Stuart Logan, Elizabeth Monck, Marie-Louise Newell, Maybelle Tatman, Andrew Tomkins, Pat Tookey.

We have also been helped by: Bev Botting, Vera Carstairs, Susan Cole, Issy Cole-Hamilton, Jacky Cooper, Anna Coote, Jean Coussins, George Davey Smith, Karen Dunnell, Aneez Esmail, Eileen Goddard, Jean Golding, Ann Johnson, Heather Joshi, Kath Kiernan, Alison Macfarlane, Hugh Markowe, Albert Osborne, Peter Phillimore, Barry Pless, Aubrey Sheiham, F. M. Sullivan, Christina Victor, Action on Smoking and Health, Baby Milk Action, Child Accident Prevention Trust, Child Poverty Action Group, Maternity Alliance, National Children's Bureau.

Finally, we thank the Wolfson Foundation for its generous financial support, North West Thames Regional Health Authority for seconding Maggie Barker to this project and the Institute of Child Health, London, where the work was carried out.

Any errors or omissions are of course our own.

Abbreviations

AAS	Annual Abstract of Statistics
AIDS	Acquired Immunodeficiency Syndrome
ALA	Association of London Authorities
ASH	Action on Smoking and Health
BMA	British Medical Association
BMI	body mass index
BMJ	*British Medical Journal*
Bq	Becquerel
CAPP	Committee on Accident and Poison Prevention
CAPT	Child Accident Prevention Trust
CDR	Communicable Disease Report
CEH	Committee on Environmental Hazards
CF	cystic fibrosis
CFC	chlorofluorocarbon
CHC	Community Health Council
CHES	Child Health and Education Survey
CHS	Continuous Household Survey (Northern Ireland)
CNS	central nervous system
CPAG	Child Poverty Action Group
CSA	Common Services Agency (Scottish NHS)
CSO	Central Statistical Office
DES	Department of Education and Science
DH	Department of Health
DH(NI)	Department of Health (Northern Ireland)
DHSS	Department of Health and Social Security
d.m.f.	decayed, missing or filled (teeth)
DoE	Department of the Environment
DoT	Department of Transport
DPT	diphtheria, polio and tetanus (vaccine)
DSS	Department of Social Security
DTI	Department of Trade and Industry
EC	European Community
EEC	European Economic Community
FoE	Friends of the Earth
FPHM	Faculty of Public Health Medicine
FSID	Foundation for the Study of Infant Deaths
GHS	General Household Survey
GP	general practitioner
HASS	Home Accident Surveillance System
HEA	Health Education Authority

Hib	Haemophilus influenzae b
HIV	human immunodeficiency virus
HMSO	Her Majesty's Stationary Office
HoN	Health of the Nation (DH publication)
HVA	Health Visitors' Association
ICD	International Classification of Diseases
LASS	Leisure Accident Surveillance System
MAFF	Ministry of Agriculture, Fisheries and Food
MMR	measles, mumps and rubella (vaccine)
MRC	Medical Research Council
mSv	milliSievert
NCH	National Children's Home
NFCA	National Foster Care Association
NFS	National Fitness Survey
NHS	National Health Service
NI	Northern Ireland
NRPB	National Radiological Protection Board
OECD	Organisation for Economic Cooperation and Development
OPCS	Office of Population Censuses and Surveys
PHLS	Public Health Laboratory Service
p.p.b.	parts per billion
p.p.m.	parts per million
RCGP	Royal College of General Practitioners
RCOG	Royal College of Obstetricians and Gynaecologists
RCP	Royal College of Physicians
RG	Registrar General
S(D)A	Stillbirths (Definition) Act
SED	Scottish Education Department
SHHD	Scottish Home and Health Department
SID	sudden infant death
TCDU	Tuberculosis and Chest Diseases Unit
UK	United Kingdom
USA	United States of America
WHO	World Health Organisation

Introduction

Children, Teenagers and Health is a ready-reference on the health of children and teenagers in the UK. The book aims to bring together the scattered data on child health. Data have been assembled from a wide range of sources. The topics covered range from child benefit to breast feeding, from road traffic accidents to child abuse, from asthma to AIDS.

Graphics have been used throughout to reveal trends and comparisons at a glance. Since the description of data sources has been kept to a minimum the reader is referred to the original for more detail of method and limitations.

Young people up to age 20, too often concealed within statistics for adults of working age, have been included wherever possible. The assumption that adulthood begins at 15 or 16 has become less valid. First, the period of dependency on parents has lengthened with increased time spent in full-time education, a rise in the number of unemployed school-leavers and a shortage of alternative housing. Second, children with severe chronic illness previously fatal in childhood may now survive and require continuity of services into adolescence and young adulthood. Third, younger teenagers are acquiring rights to self-determination, for example the right to consent to medical treatment. They are also adopting the risk behaviour of young adults in smoking, drinking, driving and sexual activity at an earlier age.

The geographical area is the UK, with comparison between the constituent countries of the UK where this is possible. Information is often not available, however, for the children of Northern Ireland. Where we have had to choose we have described England and Wales in more detail as they have the greatest number of children. In some cases the best available data are for Wales and Scotland. Although there are many excellent local studies we have used data on a national level wherever possible.

CHAPTER 1   Population and family

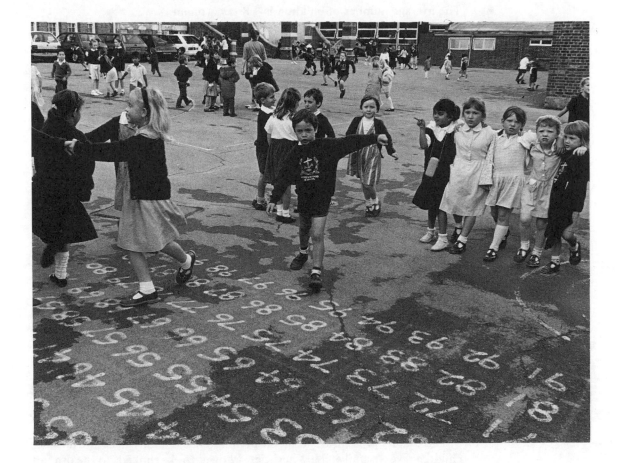

Key facts

- There are 15 million children and teenagers (age 0–19) in the UK. This age group will contribute a stable quarter of the UK population for the next fifty years.

- There are 800,000 live births a year in the UK, approximately the same number as 130 years ago.

- Eight percent of births are to teenage mothers and 9 percent are to mothers aged 35 and over (England and Wales).

- The average age of mothers at childbirth has risen to 28 years (England and Wales).

- Births outside marriage have increased to 30 percent of births. Only 8 percent of births are registered by the mother alone (England and Wales).

- The average number of children is 1.8 per woman.

- Two-thirds of children live with two parents and one or more brothers and sisters.

- A fifth of children live with a lone parent. The proportion has increased rapidly.

- Three quarters of married women with a pre-school child are in employment compared to only half of lone mothers.

- Eight percent of children under 16 belong to ethnic minority groups. The proportion has risen slowly.

Introduction

Children in the UK at the end of the twentieth century live in a population with radically different characteristics from most of the world. As a result of low birth rates and low rates of premature death the total size of the population is approaching stability.

Family structure is changing. The average number of children per woman is now less than two. The number of mothers going out to work has increased in the last decade. Births outside marriage and lone-parent families have increased. Increased adult life expectancy has meant that whereas in the past many children experienced the death of one or both parents and few knew their grandparents, today many children know both sets of grandparents and some their great-grandparents. For some children divorce and separation have replaced death as the cause of family breakdown.

This chapter presents trends in the population and family structure in which children live. Family characteristics known to be linked to health are described. Wherever possible data are shown from the child's point of view.

The population base is provided here for the chapters which follow. For example, Chapter 3 will show that infant mortality is highest among births outside marriage registered solely by the mother; Chapter 1 gives the proportion of births in this category. To understand the population impact of the increased risk of Down's syndrome in births to mothers aged 35 or more (Chapter 2) it is necessary to know what proportion of births are to mothers of that age.

Population

1.1 Population of the UK: age, 1991

Age (years)

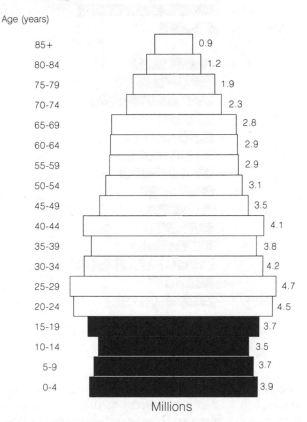

Age	Millions
85+	0.9
80-84	1.2
75-79	1.9
70-74	2.3
65-69	2.8
60-64	2.9
55-59	2.9
50-54	3.1
45-49	3.5
40-44	4.1
35-39	3.8
30-34	4.2
25-29	4.7
20-24	4.5
15-19	3.7
10-14	3.5
5-9	3.7
0-4	3.9

Millions

Source: CSO AAS 129

Total population:
57.6 million

The 15 million children and teenagers in the UK, like those in other industrialized countries, live in a population which has an age structure shaped more like a beehive than like the familiar population pyramid. As a result the total size of the population is fairly stable. Children under 15 make up a fifth of the population of the UK and of Europe. By contrast in the world as a whole a third of the population is under 15 and in some East African countries a half. At the present rate of growth it would take 300 years for the UK population to double in size whereas the population of the world is expected to double in only 40 years time (Population Reference Bureau 1992).

Children and teenagers together form a stable quarter of the population in projections for the UK to the year 2031 (CSO AAS 129). The numbers are expected to fluctuate only between 14.8 million in 1991, 15.5 million in 2001 and 15.0 million in 2031 (CSO AAS 129).

1.2 Population under 20 years old, countries and health regions of the UK, 1991

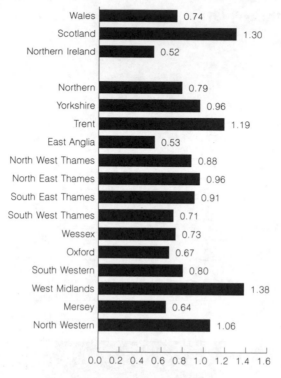

Source: CSO AAS 129

Millions

The fourteen Regional Health Authorities in England, and the countries of Wales, Scotland and Northern Ireland, have responsibility for the health of numbers of children and teenagers that ranged in 1991 from 1.38 million in the West Midlands to 0.52 million in Northern Ireland. There is even greater variation in the numbers in the next layer of authorities, the District Health Authorities and Health Boards. Boundaries are changing rapidly.

The proportion of the population under 20 years of age is higher in Northern Ireland (33 percent) than in Scotland (26 percent) or in England and Wales (25 percent) (CSO AAS 129). There is little variation among the Health Regions of England.

4

1.3 Projected change in population under 20 years old: countries and health regions of the UK, 1989–2011

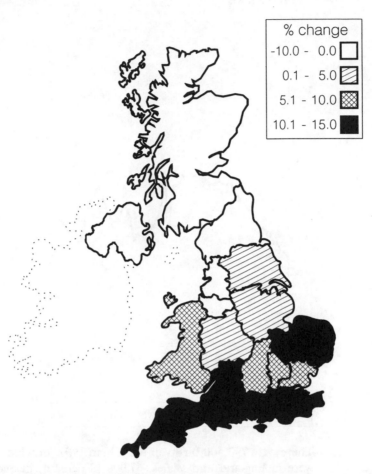

% change
-10.0 - 0.0
0.1 - 5.0
5.1 - 10.0
10.1 - 15.0

Source: OPCS PP3/8;
CSO AAS 128

Projected changes in the size of the population under age 20 vary across the UK. In the years 1989–2011 the largest increase is expected in South West Thames and the largest decrease in Northern Ireland.

At Health District level in England the largest increases in the number of children under 15 are projected for non-metropolitan areas, particularly New Towns (projected changes in the population under age 20 are not given). The expected changes range from +58 percent in Milton Keynes to −18 percent in Central Manchester (OPCS PP3/8).

Births

Throughout this chapter 'births' refers to live births only, except where live and stillbirths are specified.

1.4   Trend in births 1838–1991, England and Wales

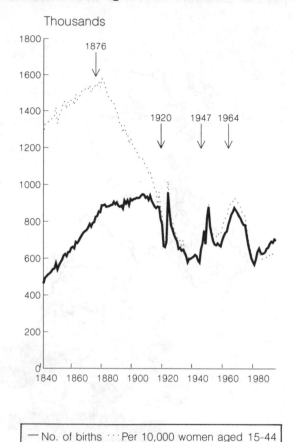

Thousands

Source: OPCS FM1

— No. of births   ⋯ Per 10,000 women aged 15-44

There were 792,500 births in the UK in 1991, of which 699,200 (88 percent) were in England and Wales, 67,000 (8 percent) in Scotland and 26,300 (3 percent) in Northern Ireland (OPCS Population Trends 69). Stillbirths made up 5 per 1000 live and stillbirths (CSO AAS 129). From 1 October 1992 the recorded number of stillbirths is likely to increase slightly following a change in the legal definition of stillbirth from a minimum gestational age of 28 weeks to 24 weeks (Stillbirth Definition Act 1992).

The number of births in England and Wales is at the same level now as 130 years ago. As a result of the decrease in family size the fertility rate (births per 1000 women aged 15–44) is less than half the level in 1860. The rate has been shown per 10,000 women aged 15–44 on Figure 1.4 for comparison. The rate fell steeply from a high point in 1876 until the First World War. Since that time the birth rate and the number of births fell sharply during the two world wars and the Great Depression of the 1930s, with steep increases immediately after the two wars. The number of births rises and falls in cycles of a generation (about 28 years) as children born in one 'bulge' become parents in the next.

In the ten years to 1991 UK births were at their highest in 1990, with 799,000 births (CSO AAS 129).

Boys are at greater risk of death than girls throughout childhood and adolescence (see Chapters 2 and 4) but more boys than girls are born. In the UK, for every 100 female births there are 105 males (CSO AAS 129).

Babies born in multiple births are at increased risk of dying in their first year. Although multiple births remain rare, the number increased steadily during the last decade, probably due to an increase in fertility treatment. In 1980 in England and Wales 9.8 per 1000 maternities resulted in multiple births. A maternity is a pregnancy ending in one or more live or stillbirths. By 1990 the rate was 11.6 per 1000 (OPCS FM1/19).

1.5   Births: age of parents, England and Wales 1991

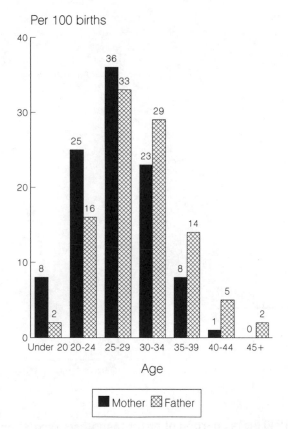

Per 100 births

Source: OPCS FM1/20

Age of father available for 92 percent of births

Child health is related to parental age. Babies born to mothers younger than 20 or older than 35 have an increased risk of dying in their first year (see Chapter 2). Children of young parents are more likely to be poor (Chapter 3) and to be exposed to passive smoking (Chapter 4). Children of older fathers are more likely to be exposed to heavy drinking (Chapter 5).

7

Of births in England and Wales in 1991, 8 percent were to mothers under 20 and 9 percent were to mothers aged 35 or more. The father's age is known for births within marriage and for births outside marriage registered jointly by both parents: 92 percent of births. Of babies where the father's age was recorded, only 2 percent had fathers who were less than 20 years old, whereas 21 percent had fathers aged 35 or more.

The proportion of births to young mothers was higher in Scotland and lower in Northern Ireland (RG Scotland 1991; DHSS N Ireland 1992).

1.6 Trend in age of mother at childbirth, England and Wales 1940–91

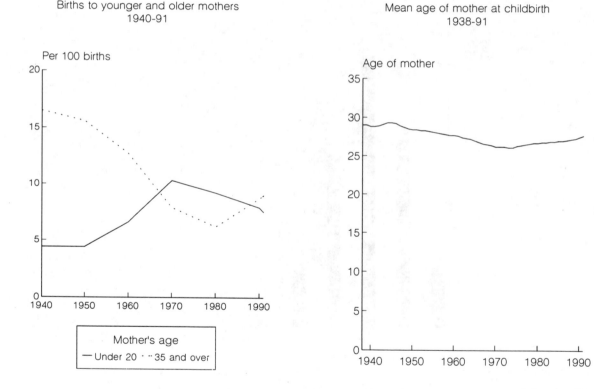

Births to younger and older mothers 1940-91

Mean age of mother at childbirth 1938-91

Source: OPCS FM1; Population Trends

Since 1940 the proportion of births to mothers aged 35 or more fell until 1980 before rising again. Conversely the proportion of births to mothers under 20 increased steeply up until 1970 before falling. The trend was similar in Scotland, but less clear in Northern Ireland.

The mean age of mothers at childbirth is 27.7 in England and Wales, slightly lower in Scotland and slightly higher in Northern Ireland.

1.7   Trend in births outside marriage, England and Wales 1977–91

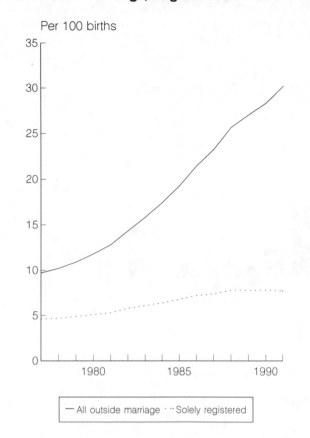

Per 100 births

Source: OPCS FM1;
Population Trends

— All outside marriage ···Solely registered

The risk of a baby dying in the first year increases with the distance of the father's relationship from the mother and baby as indicated by his status on the birth registration. Births within marriage (70 percent in 1991) have the lowest mortality, followed by births jointly registered by the mother and father living at the same address (16 percent), and births jointly registered by both parents living at different addresses (6 percent). The risk of infant death is greatest in births registered by only one parent (8 percent). (See Chapter 3.)

The proportion of births outside marriage increased steeply from 5 percent in 1960 to 30 percent in 1991. Since 1977 data have been available subdividing registrations outside marriage into those registered jointly and sole registrations. Joint registrations have been further subdivided since 1983 by whether the father gave the same or a different address from the mother.

Almost as high a proportion of births are outside marriage in Scotland (29 percent in 1991), with a lower proportion in Northern Ireland (19 percent in 1990). Among the Health Regions of England the proportion ranges from 35 percent in Merseyside to 24 percent in Oxford.

1.8 Birth registration: mother's age, England and Wales 1991

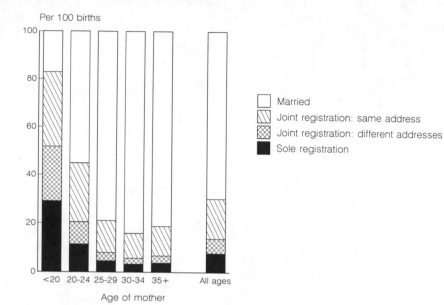

Per 100 births

Married

Joint registration: same address

Joint registration: different addresses

Sole registration

Age of mother

Source: OPCS FM1/20

1.9 Birth order, England and Wales 1990

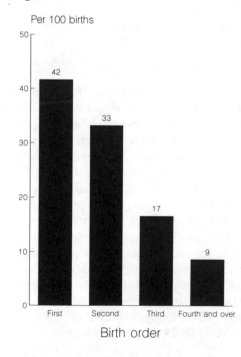

Per 100 births

Birth order

Source: Cooper and
Jones 1992

Sole registrations decline with increasing maternal age from 29 percent of all births to teenage mothers to 3 percent of births to mothers aged 30–34. Births to teenage mothers are registered within marriage (17 percent), joint registration from the same address (31 percent), joint registration from different addresses (23 percent) and sole registration (29 percent). Of births outside marriage, 21 percent are to teenage mothers, 37 percent to mothers aged 20–24 and 25 percent to mothers aged 25–29.

Using data from the OPCS General Household Survey, it has been estimated that 42 percent of all births are first births (Cooper and Jones 1992). First births have a higher risk of perinatal death (see Chapter 2).

Family structure

1.10   Trend in total fertility, England and Wales 1924–91

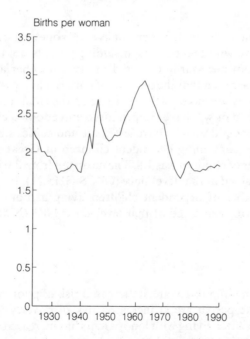

Source: OPCS FM1;
Population Trends

Children's health and development are linked to family size. For example, infant mortality is higher among third and fourth children (without taking other factors into account), and children from large families are likely to be smaller in stature (see Chapter 2).

Total fertility is the number of births a woman is likely to have if current fertility in the population continues throughout her child-bearing years. Women in England and Wales are likely to have an average of 1.8 births. The averages are 1.7 births in Scotland and 2.2 in Northern Ireland (CSO AAS 29). In England and Wales the average fluctuated between 1924 and 1991 from a maximum of 2.9 children in 1964 to a minimum of 1.7 in 1977.

1.11 Children: type of family, Great Britain 1990

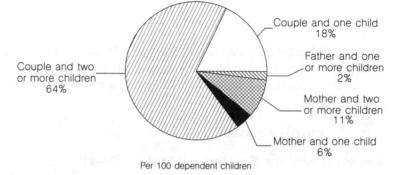

Source: OPCS GHS 21

Per 100 dependent children

Of all dependent children, 75 percent live with one or more other children and 82 percent live with two parents, including parents not legally married. (The parents are not necessarily the child's natural mother and father.)

It should be noted that the number of children living in a family at the time of the survey is not necessarily the same as the total number of children the mother has had or will have. Stepchildren and adopted children are included, whereas older children who have left home and babies still to be born are not.

In families containing dependent children in Great Britain in 1989, the mean number of children was 1.8. The mean fell from 2.0 in 1971 to 1.8 in 1981 and has remained at that level since (OPCS GHS 21). In Northern Ireland the average number of dependent children living at home was higher, at 2.2 children, having remained at that level since 1983 (N Ireland CHS 1992).

Children living in poverty are at increased risk of poor health; children living with only one parent are at increased risk of poverty (see Chapter 3). The number of children living with lone parents has increased rapidly, in particular the number living with mothers who have never married.

The estimated number of dependent children living in lone parent families in Great Britain doubled from 1.0 million in 1971 to 1.9 million in 1989 (Haskey 1991). The children increased from 8 percent of all dependent children in 1972 to 19 percent in 1990 (OPCS GHS 21).

1.12 Children in lone parent families, Great Britain

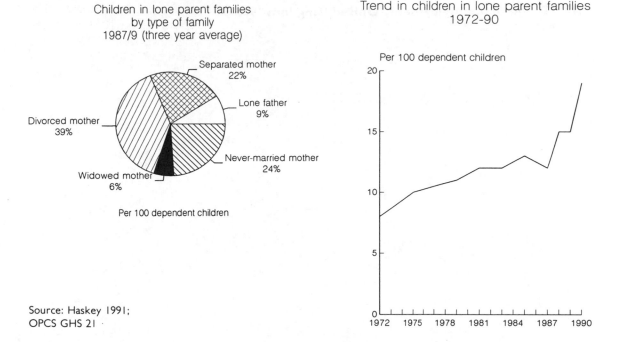

Children in lone parent families
by type of family
1987/9 (three year average)

Separated mother
22%

Lone father
9%

Divorced mother
39%

Never-married mother
24%

Widowed mother
6%

Per 100 dependent children

Trend in children in lone parent families
1972-90

Per 100 dependent children

Source: Haskey 1991;
OPCS GHS 21

Children with lone parents were more likely to have a divorced mother than any other type of lone parent, but the steepest increase has been in never-married mothers. Their number rose from 90,000 in 1971 to 360,000 in 1989, an increase of 300 percent. The rise in divorced mothers was also high (217 percent), whereas separated mothers increased by 23 percent and the number of widowed lone mothers fell by 42 percent.

Never-married mothers tend to be younger and are more likely to have a pre-school child, both factors reducing their earning capacity. Over half are aged under 25 and a quarter have a child under five years old. As would be expected, however, they also have fewer children to support. Of the children of never-married mothers, 74 percent are the only child at home. Never-married mothers are also six times more likely than divorced women to be living with their parents. In Northern Ireland lone parents head a similar proportion of all families with dependent children, 19 percent in 1990/1 (N Ireland CHS 1992).

The rapid decline in maternal mortality has reduced the risk of a baby losing its mother at birth or of an older child's mother dying in pregnancy or childbirth. The maternal mortality rate in the UK dropped from 471 per 100,000 live births in 1900 through 88 in 1950 to 8 in 1990 (CSO AAS 128). Increased overall adult life expectancy has reduced the risk of a child losing either parent through death.

13

Unemployed parents

1.13 Trend in unemployment, United Kingdom 1976–91

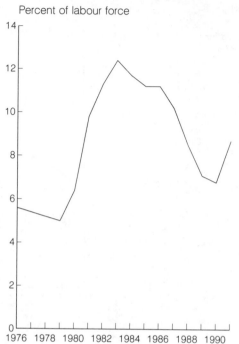

Percent of labour force

Source: CSO Social
Trends 23

Over half of children living in poverty live in a family where the head of the household is unemployed (see Chapter 3). The various definitions of unemployment are consistent in showing a peak in the early 1980s and a steep upturn in the early 1990s. Numbers of long-term unemployed (12 months or longer) decreased in the UK from 1.3 million at April 1985 to 0.8 million at April 1992 (*Working Brief* 1992). Long-term trends in unemployment are complicated by numerous changes in definitions used in the Department of Employment's statistics.

The percentage of the male workforce unemployed ranged from 7.5 percent in East Anglia to 17.8 percent in Northern Ireland, using data on numbers claiming benefit. Fathers with three or more children are twice as likely as fathers with only one child to be without paid work. In 1991 in Great Britain, among fathers with three or more children an estimated 6 percent were unemployed and 10 percent were economically inactive (neither employed nor seeking work). Among fathers with one child 4 percent were unemployed and 4 percent were economically inactive (OPCS GHS 21).

1.14 Percentage of the male workforce unemployed and claiming benefit: UK standard regions 1991

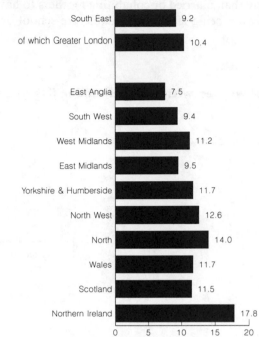

South East	9.2
of which Greater London	10.4
East Anglia	7.5
South West	9.4
West Midlands	11.2
East Midlands	9.5
Yorkshire & Humberside	11.7
North West	12.6
North	14.0
Wales	11.7
Scotland	11.5
Northern Ireland	17.8

Source: *Employment Gazette* October 1992

1.15 Mothers without employment*: marital status and age of youngest child

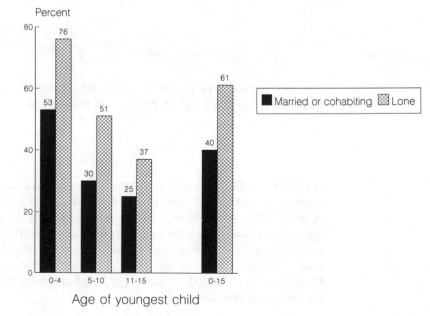

Percent

■ Married or cohabiting ▩ Lone

Age of youngest child

Age of youngest child	Married or cohabiting	Lone
0-4	53	76
5-10	30	51
11-15	25	37
0-15	40	61

Source: *Employment Gazette* October 1992

*Unemployed or economically inactive

15

Mothers' earnings are an essential protection against child poverty; for most children with lone mothers they are the only defence. However, lone mothers are less likely than married or cohabiting mothers to have paid employment, the main reason being lack of affordable pre-school or school holiday day care.

1.16 Trend in employment of women with children under five years old, Great Britain 1978–89

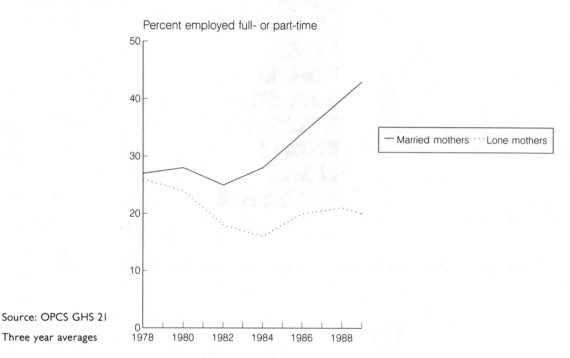

The gap between the proportion of married women and lone mothers in employment with a child under five has widened in the last decade.

In the UK less than one in five of lone mothers with a child under five years old is employed, either full-time or part-time, the third lowest figure in the EC (Cohen 1990). More lone mothers would be able to work if there were sufficient day care provision and if benefit rules made it worthwhile, but local authorities provide enough day nursery places for only 2 percent of children under three years old. In contrast, 20 percent of French and 48 percent of Danish children under three have a publicly funded day nursery place (Labour Research Department 1991).

1.17 Employment of lone mothers with a child under five years old, European Community 1988

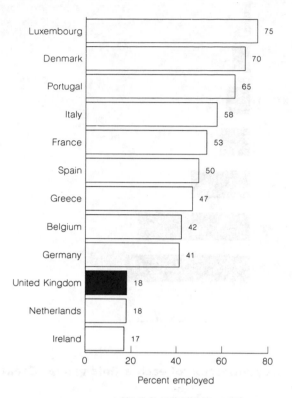

Source: Cohen 1990
from Eurostat data

Children in ethnic minorities

Health and disease vary among the children of different ethnic groups in the UK, with some minority groups having better and some worse health than the majority white population (see Chapter 3). In Great Britain in 1989/91 an estimated 8 percent of the child population under 16 years old, or 1.3 million children, were considered by their parents to belong to an ethnic minority. The largest single group is Indian (2.1 percent of all children).

The proportion of ethnic minorities in the population of all ages is highest in London and other conurbations. In the London Borough of Brent 27 percent of the all-age population belong to ethnic minorities (Haskey 1990).

National data on ethnic group have come until recently from OPCS sample surveys: the Labour Force Survey and the General Household Survey. For the first time in 1991 the Census included a question on the ethnic group to which people 'consider they belong'. The categories are White, Black-Caribbean, Black-African, Black-Other, Indian, Pakistani, Bangladeshi, Chinese and Other (Registrar General for England 1991).

17

1.18 Ethnic minority children as a proportion of all children, Great Britain 1989–91

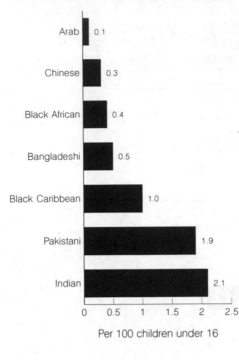

Arab 0.1
Chinese 0.3
Black African 0.4
Bangladeshi 0.5
Black Caribbean 1.0
Pakistani 1.9
Indian 2.1

Per 100 children under 16

Source: OPCS LFS 9

1.19 Children under 16 as a proportion of each ethnic group, Great Britain 1989–91

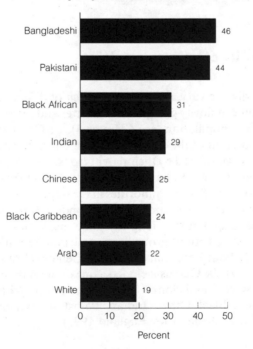

Bangladeshi 46
Pakistani 44
Black African 31
Indian 29
Chinese 25
Black Caribbean 24
Arab 22
White 19

Percent

Source: OPCS LFS 9

Family structure varies with ethnic group. Bangladeshi and Pakistani children have more siblings and fewer grandparents in this country than White children: Caribbean children have fewer siblings and are more likely to live with a lone mother. Children under 16 form nearly half the Bangladeshi and Pakistani populations compared to only a fifth of the White population. The average number of dependent children at home was 3.2 and 3.0 for Bangladeshi and Pakistani families compared to 2.1 for Indian, 1.8 for White and 1.7 for Caribbean families in Great Britain in 1987/9 (Haskey 1991). In the Bangladeshi and Pakistani populations there were as yet few people aged over 65.

The proportion of children living with only one parent ranged from 49 percent of Caribbean children through 15 percent of White children, to less than 10 percent of Indian, Pakistani or Bangladeshi children (Haskey 1991).

Of the ethnic minority population aged under 25 years 80 percent were born in the UK (OPCS GHS; personal communication).

Discussion

In Chapter 1 several problems with official data have become apparent, and these continue throughout the book. They stem mainly from definitions, categories and methods of analysis maintained to permit comparison with the past, despite rapid changes in the significance of age, family structure, gender roles and ethnic origin. A note on the history and the present form of official statistics is included at the end of the book.

There is widespread inconsistency in official publications about the appropriate age-break in mid-teens for presenting data by age group, some sources using the ages 10–14 and 15–19, and others using 10–15 and 16–19. The argument for 10–15 seems to be that legal status changes at the sixteenth birthday in some respects, for example a young woman's ability to consent to sexual intercourse. The legal status of an adult is acquired piecemeal, however, at various ages for various rights and responsibilities. Laws change, moreover, as in the raising of the school-leaving age. For comparison over time, between countries and with other five-year age groups, the use of 10–14 and 15–19 is preferred. At least UK authors are not often guilty of the US practice of describing children only by their school year, prohibiting international comparison. Young people aged 15–19 are sometimes included with younger children under the definition of 'dependent children', which creates difficulties in comparison over time and between countries, as the proportion of dependent 15–19 year olds varies. In other data the age group 15–19 is invisible, included with the entire population of working age.

The rapid increase in births outside marriage and lone parenthood, in cohabitation and in women's equality requires changes to official methods of recording and analysing data. 'Birth order' as presently defined is limited to births within marriage. Thus, a first child within marriage is classified as a first birth even if the mother has had previous children outside marriage. Children born outside marriage are not allocated a birth order, and as they form a growing proportion of births data are increasingly distorted by this practice. The Government has proposed legislation to record the same information for all births (Secretary of State for Health 1990).

Births outside marriage registered by the mother alone and children living with lone mothers cannot be assigned a social class (defined by father's occupation) and are thus excluded from most social class analyses (Cooper and Botting 1992). Cohabiting couples are sometimes but not always counted as married. Analysis by household has also become less informative when a third of households (of all ages) are people living on their own. Married women (and their children) are usually allocated the social class of their husband, although their own occupation may be in another class.

As regards ethnic group, data on birth and death are still available only by country of birth, or in the case of an infant by country of birth of the mother. This is of decreasing relevance as ethnic minorities become established in the UK.

Finally, there is a constant problem in extracting data from the perspective of the child where the household is the unit of analysis. How many children are in households where the father is unemployed? How many children, as compared to families, are homeless? Most existing data cannot answer these questions.

References

Publications other than routine data series

Cohen, B. (1990) *Caring for Children: the 1990 Report*. London, Family Policy Studies Centre.

Cooper, J. and Botting, B. (1992) 'Analysing fertility and infant mortality by mother's social class as defined by occupation', *OPCS Population Trends* 70: 15–21.

Cooper, J. S. and Jones, C. (1992) 'Estimates of the numbers of first, second, third and higher order births', *OPCS Population Trends* 70: 8–14.

Craig, J. (1992) 'Recent fertility trends in Europe', *OPCS Population Trends* 68: 20–5.

Department of Health (1992) *Children in Care in England and Wales, March 1990*. London, DH.

Employment Gazette (1992) London, Employment Department, October, S20–4.

Haskey, J. (1990) 'The ethnic minority populations resident in private households – estimates by county and metropolitan district of England and Wales', *OPCS Population Trends* 63: 22–35.

Haskey, J. (1991) 'Estimated numbers and demographic characteristics of one-parent families in Great Britain', *OPCS Population Trends* 65: 35–43.

Labour Research Department (1991) *Bargaining Report III*. London, LRD.

Northern Ireland Continuous Household Survey (1992) Belfast, Policy and Planning Research Unit, CHS 1/92.

Population Reference Bureau (1992) *World Population Data Sheet*. New York, PRB.

Registrar General for England (1991) *Census Form for Private Households*. London, HMSO.

Secretary of State for Health (1990) *Registration: Proposals for Change*. London, HMSO.

Working Brief (1992) London, Unemployment Unit and Youth Aid, June, 18.

Routine data series

Office of Population Censuses and Surveys:
    OPCS DH3 Mortality Statistics: Perinatal and Infant
    OPCS FM1 Birth Statistics
    OPCS FM2 Marriage and Divorce Statistics
    OPCS PP2 Population Projections
    OPCS PP3 Sub-national Population Projections
    OPCS GHS General Household Survey
    OPCS LFS Labour Force Survey
    Population Trends
Central Statistical Office:
    CSO Annual Abstract of Statistics (AAS)
    CSO Regional Trends
    CSO Social Trends
Registrar General for Northern Ireland:
    RG N Ireland Annual Reports
Registrar General for Scotland:
    RG Scotland Annual Reports

CHAPTER 2

Mortality and morbidity

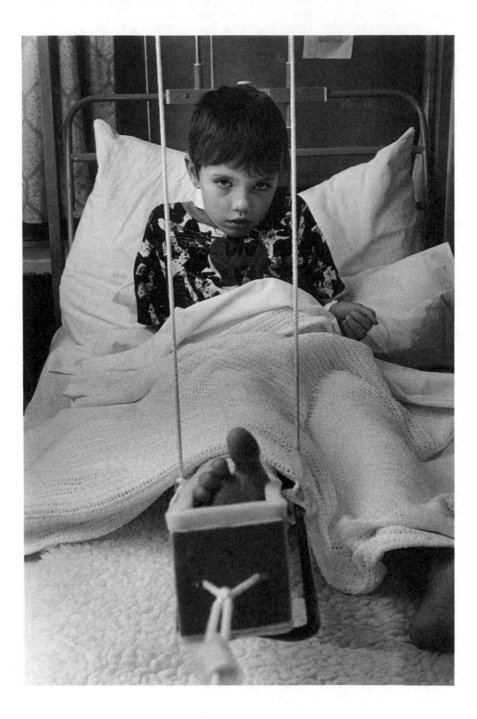

Key facts

- UK mortality under the age of 20 years has fallen by over 90 percent during the twentieth century.

- Over half of deaths under 20 years occur in infancy, a third in the first month of life. The main causes of infant death are congenital anomaly (24 percent), sudden infant death (19 percent) and prematurity (17 percent).

- Low birthweight increases the risk of mortality and morbidity (for example cerebral palsy). The proportion of low weight babies surviving is increasing.

- Prenatal screening has reduced the prevalence of congenital disorders (for example spina bifida) at birth, while improved treatment has increased survival after birth.

- Injuries cause 47 percent of deaths among 1–19 year olds, increasing in importance from 24 percent of all deaths aged 1–4 to 60 percent of deaths aged 15–19. Eighty percent of fatal injuries are accidental.

- Chronic illness in under-16s, including respiratory disease and diabetes, has increased over the past 20 years. Fourteen per cent of children under 16 have a longstanding illness and 3 percent have a disability (Great Britain 1990).

- Many children are on child protection registers or in local authority care because of physical or sexual abuse, neglect or deprivation, but the true extent of these problems is unknown.

Introduction

This chapter provides a summary of childhood and teenage mortality and morbidity in the UK, showing the numbers experiencing different types of illness and disability, and thus the relative need for prevention and care. The term *mortality* is used throughout to refer to death rates; that is, the number of deaths as a proportion of the population of the relevant age. The term *morbidity* covers all forms of ill-health. Along with the demographic overview in Chapter 1, this chapter gives the background to the presentation of socioeconomic, environmental and behavioural factors in subsequent chapters. It is in three sections.

'*Mortality overview*' covers mortality time-trends, age distribution, demographic factors and the principal causes of death. '*Morbidity overview*' provides direct evidence on ill-health and disability in the population under 20 years old, and indirect evidence from use of health and social services. '*Selected conditions*' gives a sketch of some epidemiological features of a range of causes of death and illness in childhood. Topics have been selected for their public health importance, and differ widely in the severity of the condition and numbers affected.

Measuring health

Health is multi-dimensional and difficult to define; its absence is easier to measure than its presence. Mortality is the most commonly used index of ill-health, and data on deaths in the UK are, on the whole, reliably recorded through the system of death registration. However, death is an extreme measure and makes up only one small part of the total health experience of the population; less than 0.1 percent of the population under 20 years of age die per year.

It has been estimated that at least 3 percent of children and young people suffer from a permanent disability. The most recent nationally representative surveys of chronic illness and disability among children are the OPCS General Household Survey (GHS) (OPCS GHS 1990) and the OPCS Disability Survey (Bone and Meltzer 1989). Both surveys rely on parents' reporting of their children's health. The GHS has estimated 'chronic sickness' among children living in private households in Great Britain annually since 1971. Parents are asked of children under 16, 'Do any of your children have any longstanding illness, disability or infirmity?' Longstanding is defined as 'anything that has troubled them over a period of time or that is likely to affect them over a period of time'. Illness which is not only longstanding but also limits activity is defined by a further question, 'Does this illness or disability limit the child's activities in any way?' In 1988–9 only, replies were categorized by diagnostic group (ICD9; see Glossary). Young people aged 16–19 answer similar questions for themselves.

In 1991, for the first time, the Census included a question on health, asking of the entire population, 'Does the person have any long-term illness, health problem or handicap which limits his/her daily activities or the work he/she can do?' Survey data obtained in this manner are subject to the limitation that responses are influenced by individual perceptions. Perceived 'limitation of activity' will vary greatly according to past experience, demands and expectations.

The OPCS Disability Survey in 1985–6 was also based on parents' reports for their children, and on teenagers aged 16–19 responding for themselves. In contrast to the GHS, this survey included the small proportion of children (over five years old only) in institutions, for whom the staff responded. Disabilities were categorized by diagnostic group (ICD9) and by function, for instance reduced ability to see, hear or walk (International Classification of Impairments, Disabilities and Handicaps).

Measuring the great mass of temporary and less serious illness, which can cause suffering to children and their families, is even more problematic. The GHS collects some data on acute sickness (restriction of the individual's normal activities) and recent use of health services. These data are useful because they are obtained from a large sample of the population, and show sufficiently consistent patterns to make them useful for comparison over time and by age, sex and social factors. They provide some indication of the total burden of ill-health, including colds, headaches, stomach upsets and minor injuries, as well as serious problems, some of which never come to the attention of the health service.

Information on children's health is also available from the three national birth cohort studies, which followed children born in Great Britain in one week in 1946, 1958 and 1970 and monitored their health at various ages. In contrast to the GHS, information was collected for a wide range of specific conditions, by both interviews and medical examinations, and for the same children over time (Butler and Golding 1986; Wadsworth 1987; Power 1992). While the birth cohort studies provide valuable data on a national sample of children, they will not necessarily continue to reflect contemporary problems. It is hoped that new surveys planned by the Department of Health will rectify this through regular child health monitoring.

National registers such as those for congenital anomalies and cancer collect valuable data, but these need to be used with care. The completeness and accuracy of reporting depend on the commitment of local personnel and the efficiency of data collection mechanisms. Changes in completeness of reporting, definitions or criteria for inclusion may complicate monitoring of trends over time.

The difficulty of measuring health sometimes makes it necessary to depend on the use of health services as a 'proxy' measure, but it is important to recognize the limitations of this for measuring the actual health of the population.

Hospital information systems at present are designed to record hospital activity, not the health of individuals or of the population. Because hospital statistics count discharges or episodes, one person admitted to hospital twice cannot be distinguished from two people admitted once each; nor can a stay in hospital of one day easily be distinguished from one of a month. Changes in hospital activity over time may not reflect real changes in health, since criteria for referral or admission may vary, depending on medical knowledge and availability of treatment. Comparison between different areas is also complicated by the fact that the availability of hospital beds or other resources is itself a major determinant of admissions, irrespective of the level of illness in the population.

Trends in the admission of children to hospital in recent years have been affected by increasing awareness of the benefits, both psychological (Thornes 1990; DH 1991a) and economic (Audit Commission 1991), of day surgery and home care. Average length of stay in hospital (England and Wales) has fallen. In 1974 this was 7.4 days of children 0–4 years old and 5.9 days for children 5–14 years old; in 1985, 4.8 and 4.1 days; and in 1988–9, 3.7 and 3.8 days (OPCS MB4/29). At the same time, the proportion of admissions which are re-admissions has increased (Henderson et al. 1989; Hill 1989).

Cause of death and many other health-related data are classified according to the International Classification of Diseases (ICD9). In the case of stillbirths and neonatal deaths, both fetal and maternal causes can be recorded. All references to causes of neonatal death in this chapter are based on main fetal cause only. Deaths at subsequent ages are classified to a single cause.

Mortality overview

This section outlines time-trends in deaths under 20, the age distribution and principal causes of mortality. Mortality statistics are collected through death registrations and published by the Office of Population Censuses and Surveys (OPCS) for England and Wales and the respective Registrars General for Scotland and Northern Ireland.

Infant deaths (deaths under one year of age) are conventionally divided into perinatal (stillbirths and under one week of age), neonatal (in the first four weeks of life) and postneonatal (four weeks and under one year). Stillbirths are defined as fetal deaths after 28 weeks of gestation; from October 1992 this is 24 weeks (S(D)A 1992). When a mortality rate is calculated, stillbirths and perinatal deaths are per 1000 live and stillbirths; neonatal, postneonatal and infant deaths are per 1000 live births only. After one year, mortality rates are based on the estimated population in the relevant age group.

2.1   Trend in infant mortality 1841–5 to 1986–90, England and Wales

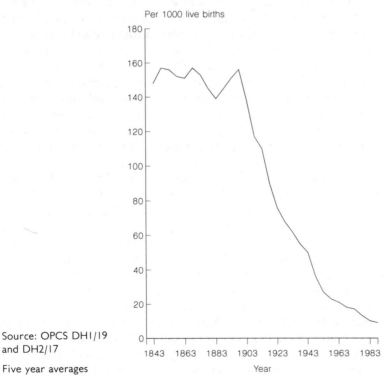

Source: OPCS DH1/19 and DH2/17

Five year averages

2.2 Trend in mortality under 20 years 1841–5 to 1986–90, England and Wales

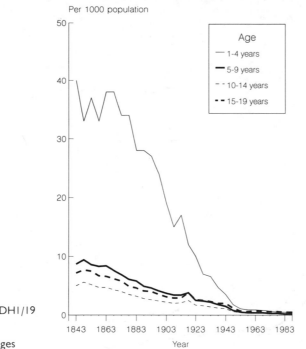

Per 1000 population

Source: OPCS DH1/19
and DH2/17

Five year averages

2.3 Trend in infant mortality 1941–5 to 1991, England and Wales

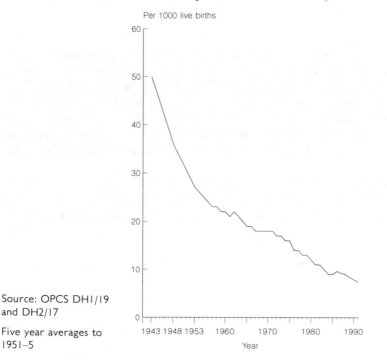

Per 1000 live births

Source: OPCS DH1/19
and DH2/17

Five year averages to
1951–5

2.4 Trend in mortality under 20 years 1941–5 to 1990, England and Wales

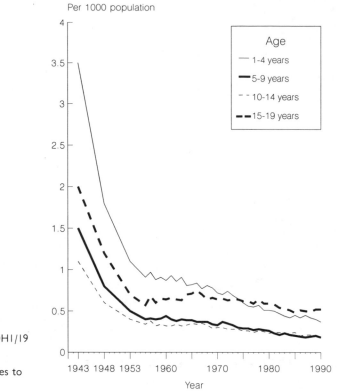

Per 1000 population

Source: OPCS DH1/19
and DH2/17

Five year averages to
1951–5

Mortality at all ages has fallen steadily over the last 150 years in response to improved living conditions, diet and sanitation, birth control, advances in medical science and the availability of health care. Infant mortality, long regarded as an important indicator of the national health, was 148 per 1000 live births in England and Wales in 1841–5, 50 in 1941–5, and reached 7.9 in 1990 (OPCS DH1/19, DH2/17; OPCS Monitor DH3 91/2). Mortality at all ages from 1 to 19 years have been below 1 per 1000 since 1956 (OPCS DH1/19, DH2/17).

Infant mortality in Scotland was 68 per 1000 in 1941–5 and 7.7 in 1990 (RG Scotland 1990). In Northern Ireland, infant mortality in 1990 was 7.5 per 1000 (RG N Ireland 1991). Overall mortality at 1–19 years is similar throughout the UK.

2.5   Deaths under 20 years: age, United Kingdom 1990

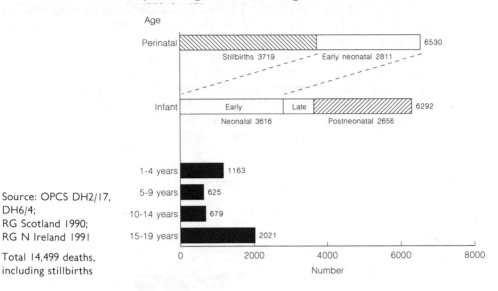

Age

Perinatal — Stillbirths 3719 — Early neonatal 2811 — 6530

Infant — Early Neonatal 3616 — Late Postneonatal 2656 — 6292

1-4 years — 1163
5-9 years — 625
10-14 years — 679
15-19 years — 2021

Number

Source: OPCS DH2/17,
DH6/4;
RG Scotland 1990;
RG N Ireland 1991

Total 14,499 deaths,
including stillbirths

2.6   Mortality under 20 years: age, United Kingdom 1990

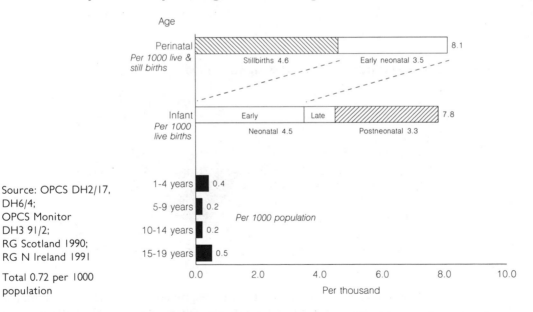

Age

Perinatal
*Per 1000 live &
still births* — Stillbirths 4.6 — Early neonatal 3.5 — 8.1

Infant
*Per 1000
live births* — Early Neonatal 4.5 — Late Postneonatal 3.3 — 7.8

1-4 years — 0.4
5-9 years — 0.2   *Per 1000 population*
10-14 years — 0.2
15-19 years — 0.5

Per thousand

Source: OPCS DH2/17,
DH6/4;
OPCS Monitor
DH3 91/2;
RG Scotland 1990;
RG N Ireland 1991

Total 0.72 per 1000
population

Death in childhood, after the age of one year, has become a relatively rare
event. In 1990 there were 4488 deaths of children and young people aged 1–19
years in the UK, 0.03 percent of the population at that age (OPCS DH2/17;

RG Scotland 1990; RG N Ireland 1991). Fifty-eight percent of all deaths under 20 years happen in infancy. The 99.2 percent of babies surviving the first year of life face a decreasing risk of death until traffic accidents take an increasing toll from age 15 onwards.

In infancy and the late teenage years, mortality in boys is higher than in girls, possibly reflecting greater vulnerability to a range of conditions, and especially a greater propensity to suffer accidental injuries. Infant mortality in the UK was 6.8 per 1000 girls and 8.8 per 1000 boys in 1990. Mortality was similar for girls and boys aged 1–14 years, but at 15–19 the rates were 0.3 for young women and 0.7 for young men (CSO AAS 128).

2.7   Causes of neonatal death, United Kingdom 1990

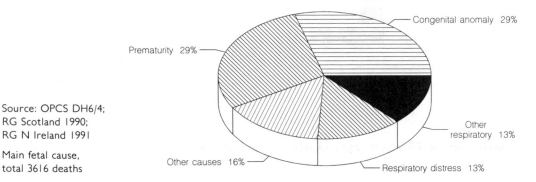

Source: OPCS DH6/4;
RG Scotland 1990;
RG N Ireland 1991

Main fetal cause,
total 3616 deaths

2.8   Causes of postneonatal death, United Kingdom 1990

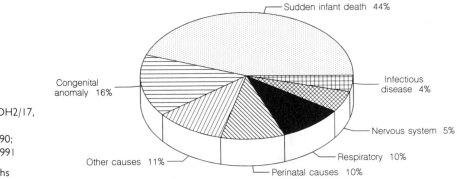

Source: OPCS DH2/17,
DH6/4;
RG Scotland 1990;
RG N Ireland 1991

Total 2656 deaths

The principal causes of neonatal death are prematurity, congenital anomalies (especially those of the central nervous system, heart and circulation) and perinatal respiratory problems (OPCS DH6/4). Between the ages of 28 days and one year, the most common cause of death is sudden infant death (SID; 'cot death').

30

2.9 Causes of infant death, United Kingdom 1990

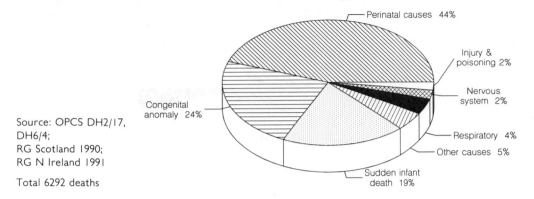

Perinatal causes 44%

Injury & poisoning 2%

Nervous system 2%

Congenital anomaly 24%

Respiratory 4%

Other causes 5%

Sudden infant death 19%

Source: OPCS DH2/17, DH6/4;
RG Scotland 1990;
RG N Ireland 1991

Total 6292 deaths

Congenital anomalies cause a quarter of deaths in infancy, and continue to cause significant mortality up to early adolescence. Perinatal causes contribute to mortality for some months after birth (OPCS DH2/17; RG Scotland 1990; RG N Ireland 1991).

2.10 Causes of death age 1–4 years, United Kingdom 1990

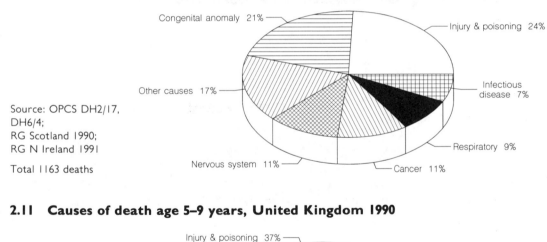

Congenital anomaly 21%

Injury & poisoning 24%

Other causes 17%

Infectious disease 7%

Source: OPCS DH2/17, DH6/4;
RG Scotland 1990;
RG N Ireland 1991

Total 1163 deaths

Nervous system 11%

Cancer 11%

Respiratory 9%

2.11 Causes of death age 5–9 years, United Kingdom 1990

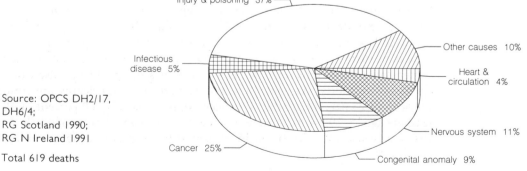

Injury & poisoning 37%

Other causes 10%

Infectious disease 5%

Heart & circulation 4%

Source: OPCS DH2/17, DH6/4;
RG Scotland 1990;
RG N Ireland 1991

Total 619 deaths

Nervous system 11%

Cancer 25%

Congenital anomaly 9%

31

2.12   Causes of death age 10–14 years, United Kingdom 1990

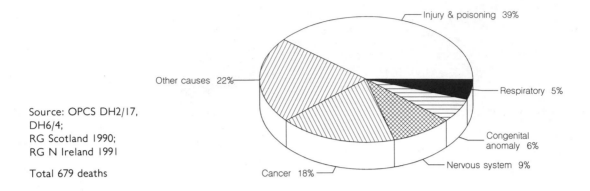

Injury & poisoning 39%

Respiratory 5%

Congenital anomaly 6%

Nervous system 9%

Cancer 18%

Other causes 22%

Source: OPCS DH2/17, DH6/4;
RG Scotland 1990;
RG N Ireland 1991

Total 679 deaths

2.13   Causes of death age 15–19 years, United Kingdom 1990

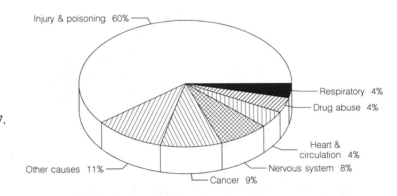

Injury & poisoning 60%

Respiratory 4%

Drug abuse 4%

Heart & circulation 4%

Nervous system 8%

Cancer 9%

Other causes 11%

Source: OPCS DH2/17, DH6/4;
RG Scotland 1990;
RG N Ireland 1991

Total 2021 deaths

After the first year of life, injuries (including poisoning) become the largest single cause of death, with a rate of 172 per million boys and 98 per million girls aged 1–4 years in 1990. In older children the importance of injuries as a cause of death is even more pronounced. Diseases of the nervous system, such as meningitis, other infectious diseases and respiratory problems, also cause significant mortality. At age 5–9 years, 37 percent of all deaths are from injuries and 25 percent are due to cancer. Injuries make up 60 percent of all deaths at age 15–19, with cancer remaining the second main cause of death. At least 4 percent of deaths in the 15–19 age group are from drug abuse (see Chapter 5).

2.14   Causes of death age 0–19 years, United Kingdom 1990

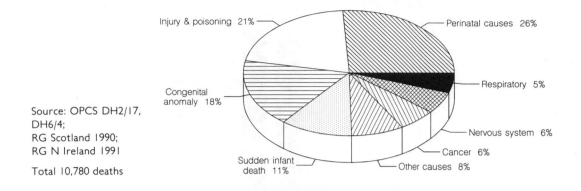

Injury & poisoning 21%

Perinatal causes 26%

Respiratory 5%

Congenital anomaly 18%

Nervous system 6%

Cancer 6%

Sudden infant death 11%

Other causes 8%

Source: OPCS DH2/17,
DH6/4;
RG Scotland 1990;
RG N Ireland 1991

Total 10,780 deaths

2.15   Causes of death age 1–19 years, United Kingdom 1990

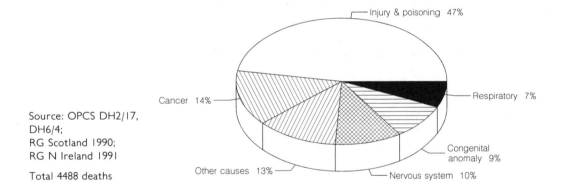

Injury & poisoning 47%

Respiratory 7%

Cancer 14%

Congenital anomaly 9%

Other causes 13%

Nervous system 10%

Source: OPCS DH2/17,
DH6/4;
RG Scotland 1990;
RG N Ireland 1991

Total 4488 deaths

If infancy is included, perinatal conditions are the largest single cause of death under 20 years of age. If infancy is excluded, the largest single cause is injury.

Low birthweight is associated with increased risk of death and illness throughout childhood (Hack *et al.* 1981; Mutch *et al.* 1986). Improved chances of survival for very low birthweight babies (under 1500 g) have therefore been accompanied by concerns about increasing morbidity in the child population (Chalmers and Mutch 1981).

2.16   Live births: birthweight, England and Wales 1990

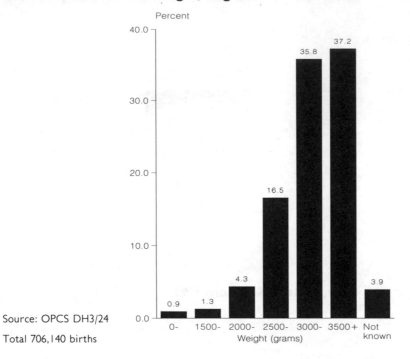

Percent

Source: OPCS DH3/24

Total 706,140 births

2.17   Infant mortality: birthweight, England and Wales 1990

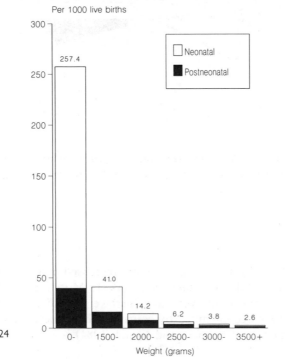

Per 1000 live births

Source: OPCS DH3/24

The current definition of low birthweight is less than 2500 g, or 5.5 *lbs*. Very low birthweight is defined as less than 1500 g, or 3.3 *lbs*. Births under 1500 g make up 0.9 percent of live births, and all those under 2500 g make up 6.5 percent (England and Wales 1990) (OPCS DH3/24).

Mortality figures for England and Wales in 1990 show that babies weighing under 1500 g at birth were 34 times more likely than babies of all weights to die in the perinatal period, 48 times more likely to die in the first four weeks of life, and 12 times more likely to die between four weeks and one year. Babies weighing under 2500 g had nine times the risk of neonatal death of all babies and four times the risk of postneonatal death (OPCS DH3/24).

2.18   Low birthweight: mother's age, England and Wales 1990

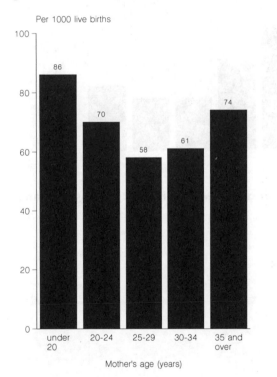

Source: OPCS DH3/24

Births under 2500 g

The distribution of births by mother's age is described in Chapter 1. Babies of mothers aged under 20 and over 35 years have the highest rates of low birthweight, perinatal and neonatal mortality (without taking parity into account). After the first four weeks of life the excess mortality in children of older women diminishes, while the postneonatal mortality in children of women aged under 20 is more than twice that in children of mothers aged 25 and upwards. Infants of younger mothers are more likely to die of respiratory conditions, infectious diseases, injuries and sudden infant death; fatal congenital anomalies are more common in infants of mothers over 35 (OPCS DH3/24).

35

2.19   Infant mortality: mother's age, England and Wales 1990

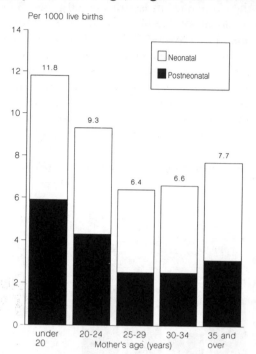

Per 1000 live births

Source: OPCS DH3/24

2.20   Infant mortality: birth order within marriage, England and Wales 1990

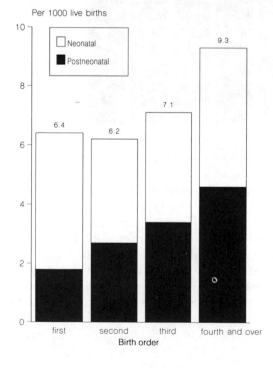

Per 1000 live births

Source: OPCS DH3/24

36

Infant mortality by birth order is available for England and Wales only for the 70 percent of births which are within marriage, and in calculating birth order only previous births within marriage are counted. The distribution of births by birth order is described in Chapter 1. With birth order so defined, infant mortality is similar for first and second births but increases thereafter. Neonatal mortality is highest in first and fourth or subsequent births, while postneonatal mortality increases steadily with birth order. The effect of excluding births outside marriage is probably to underestimate the excess mortality in first as compared to second births.

Evidence from Norway, where data permit longitudinal analysis, point to the likelihood that perinatal mortality decreases with birth order if births are grouped according to the mother's completed parity (Bakketeig and Hoffman 1979).

2.21 Infant mortality: mother's country of birth, England and Wales 1990

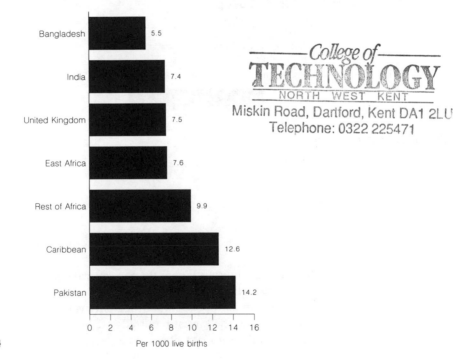

Source: OPCS DH3/24

Infant mortality in babies of mothers born in Pakistan is nearly twice that of mothers born in the UK. Infants of women born in the Caribbean also have high mortality, while infants of mothers born in Bangladesh are at lower risk (OPCS DH3/24).

Mortality in infants of ethnic minority mothers born in the UK is not available. The birth record includes mother's country of birth, but not the mother's or baby's ethnic group. In 1988–90, 5.6 percent of births in England and Wales were to mothers born in the Caribbean, Africa and Asia (OPCS

37

FM1/19). Another 1 percent were to mothers from Caribbean, African and Asian ethnic groups born in the UK (Shaw 1988). The difference between country of birth and ethnic group increases with the length of time the particular community has been settled in the UK. This means that the average age of mothers identifiable in infant mortality data as Caribbean is higher than in the population as a whole. In Scotland in 1990, 1.4 percent of births were to mothers born in the New Commonwealth and Pakistan (RG Scotland 1990).

The high infant mortality in babies of mothers born in Pakistan is partly owing to a greater frequency of congenital anomalies (see Congenital disorders). Conversely, infants whose mother was born in India, Pakistan, Bangladesh or Africa have lower rates of sudden infant death than babies whose mothers were born in the UK (Balarajan *et al.* 1989a,b). This may be because few such women smoke, and they are probably less likely to put babies to sleep face down or in a room on their own.

2.22 Infant mortality 1988–9: Europe

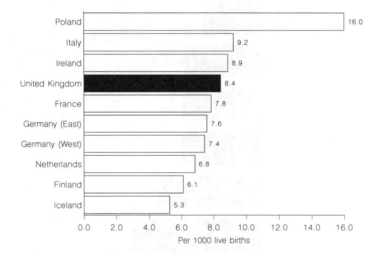

Source: WHO
Eurostat/PC
1992

UK infant mortality is higher than in several comparable Western European countries, such as France, Germany and the Netherlands (WHO Eurostat/PC 1992). Western European infant mortality is better than in most parts of the world, although the lowest reported rate (4.8 per 10000 in 1990) is in Japan (World Population Data Sheet 1992).

Morbidity overview

This section presents measures of chronic illness and disability among children, followed by measures which combine chronic and acute illness (such as GP consultations and hospital admissions). Some measures describe the children; others describe the conditions. Many ill children have more than one condition.

38

2.23   Trend in chronic illness (longstanding illness) 1972–91, Great Britain

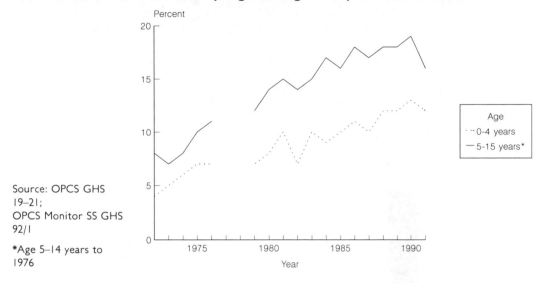

Percent

Source: OPCS GHS
19–21;
OPCS Monitor SS GHS
92/1

*Age 5–14 years to
1976

Age
··· 0-4 years
—— 5-15 years*

Year

2.24   Trend in chronic illness (limiting longstanding illness) 1972–91, Great Britain

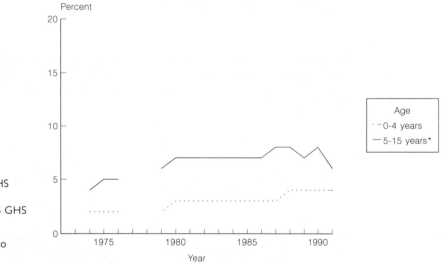

Percent

Source: OPCS GHS
19–21;
OPCS Monitor SS GHS
92/1

*Age 5–14 years to
1976

Age
··· 0-4 years
—— 5-15 years*

Year

According to the GHS the prevalence of chronic illness in childhood more than doubled between 1972 and 1991 (OPCS GHS). Although the trend over time may in part reflect changes in parents' expectations of their children's health, and greater assessment of morbidity resulting from increased access to medical care, the increase in the prevalence of chronic diseases such as asthma has been supported by other data (Anderson 1989; Burney *et al*. 1990) and respiratory disease accounts for a large proportion of reported chronic illness.

2.25 Chronic illness: age, Great Britain 1991

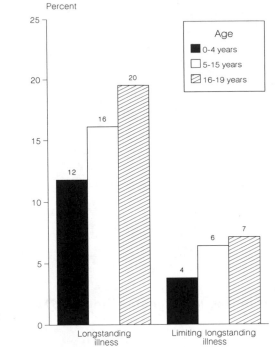

Percent

Age
- ■ 0-4 years
- □ 5-15 years
- ▨ 16-19 years

Source: OPCS GHS;
personal
communication

The prevalence of chronic illness increases with age, and it is more commonly reported in boys than in girls. In 1991 a fifth of young people aged 16–19 reported that they had a longstanding illness (OPCS GHS).

Both boys and girls aged 0–15 years with a longstanding illness had an average (mean) of 1.2 conditions per child. The most commonly reported condition was a respiratory illness, usually asthma; 78 per 1000 children – half of those with longstanding illness – had a respiratory condition. Skin complaints (eczema) and ear complaints were also frequently mentioned (OPCS GHS 20). Asthma is a major cause of chronic ill-health throughout childhood (see Respiratory conditions).

2.26 Longstanding illness age 0–15 years: type of illness, Great Britain 1989

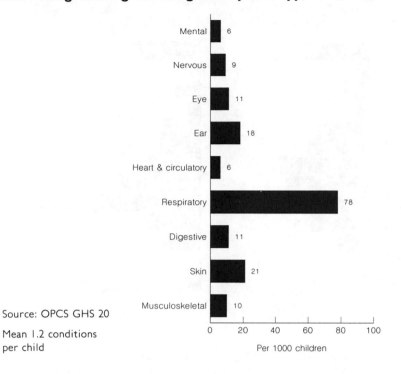

Mental 6
Nervous 9
Eye 11
Ear 18
Heart & circulatory 6
Respiratory 78
Digestive 11
Skin 21
Musculoskeletal 10

Source: OPCS GHS 20

Mean 1.2 conditions per child

Per 1000 children

2.27 Children with a disability: age and sex, Great Britain 1985–8

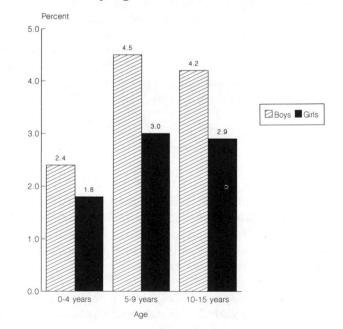

Percent

Boys Girls

0-4 years: 2.4, 1.8
5-9 years: 4.5, 3.0
10-15 years: 4.2, 2.9

Age

Source: Bone and Meltzer 1989

2.28 Disabilities: functional categories, Great Britain 1985–8

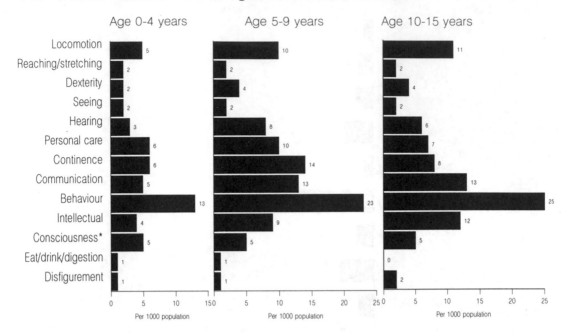

Age 0-4 years | Age 5-9 years | Age 10-15 years

Per 1000 population

Source: Bone and
Meltzer 1989

*Includes fits and
convulsions

The reported prevalence of disability is slightly lower than the GHS figure for limiting longstanding illness, with parents reporting in the Disability Survey that 3 percent of 0–15 year olds in Britain (360,000) had a disability. Of the 11 percent of disabled 5–15 year olds with the most severe disabilities, less than 1 in 20 lived in institutions. The prevalence of disability increased from the pre-school years to age 5–9, as parents became aware of disabilities when their children entered school. More boys were reported disabled than girls. Nearly two-thirds of disabled children were restricted in more than one function. The most common category of functional disability was a behavioural problem (see Mental Health) (Bone and Meltzer 1989).

The most striking difference in reported disability between under-15s and 16–19 year olds is a sudden fall in behaviour problems. This may be because of the survey methods: young people over 15 replied on their own behalf and the questions asked were slightly different. Less disability was reported by older teenagers in all categories except seeing and disfigurement (Bone and Meltzer 1989).

Another measure of disability among school-age children is the number of statements of special educational need, which define any special requirements

2.29 Disabilities age 16–19 years: functional categories, Great Britain 1985–8

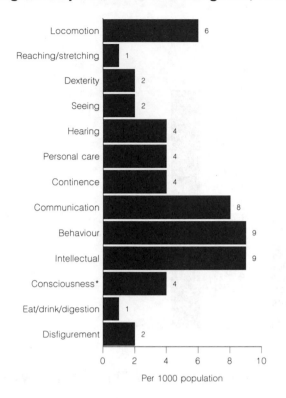

Locomotion 6
Reaching/stretching 1
Dexterity 2
Seeing 2
Hearing 4
Personal care 4
Continence 4
Communication 8
Behaviour 9
Intellectual 9
Consciousness* 4
Eat/drink/digestion 1
Disfigurement 2

0   2   4   6   8   10

Per 1000 population

Source: Bone and
Meltzer 1989

*Includes fits and
convulsions

a child has due to physical or mental disability. In 1991 there were 148,300 children aged 5–16 with such statements, or 2 percent of the population of school age in England and Wales (DES 1992). As statements imply financial commitment to provide special education, policies for issuing a statement vary between authorities and over time. The number of children with statements increased by 11 percent between January 1989 and January 1991.

The GHS also asks about short-term illness and use of health services. The proportion of children with recent illness, defined as having their normal activities restricted by illness in the past fortnight, has increased in recent years. Children under five years old are twice as likely as older children to have seen a general practitioner (GP) in the past fortnight, including consultation by telephone (OPCS GHS 21; personal communication). Many of their visits will have been for immunizations and routine check-ups, which are increasingly provided by GPs.

2.30   Illness and GP contact in the past fortnight: age, Great Britain 1990

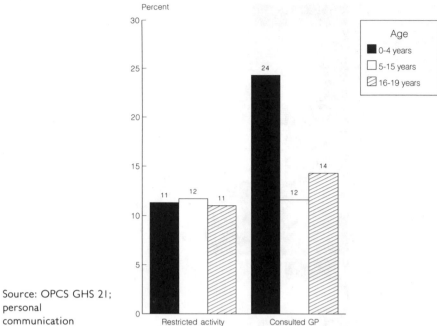

Source: OPCS GHS 21;
personal
communication

2.31   Reasons for GP consultation, age 0–4 years, England and Wales 1981–2

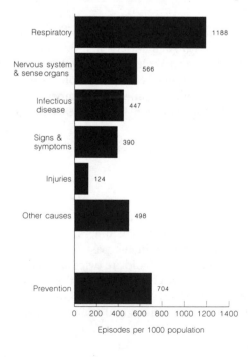

Source: OPCS MB5/1

2.32   Reasons for GP consultation, age 5–14 years, England and Wales 1981–2

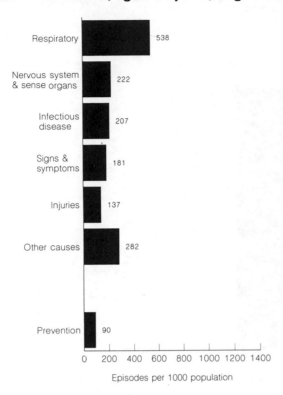

Respiratory — 538
Nervous system & sense organs — 222
Infectious disease — 207
Signs & symptoms — 181
Injuries — 137
Other causes — 282
Prevention — 90

0 200 400 600 800 1000 1200 1400

Episodes per 1000 population

Source: OPCS MB5/1

A national study of general practice in 1981–2 showed that a third of all episodes of illness in childhood in which the GP was consulted were caused by respiratory complaints. Eighteen percent of consultations by children under five years old were for routine developmental checks, immunization or other preventive care (OPCS MB5/1). The study involved some 1 percent of children under 15 in England and Wales, but may not be representative of the whole population as the GPs taking part were volunteers. A similar study took place in 1991–2.

Nearly one-tenth of all children under five years of age were admitted to hospital at least once in 1990. The proportion with a hospital stay was lower at 16–19 years and least at 5–15 years (OPCS GHS 21; personal communication).

2.33 Admission to hospital in the past year: age, Great Britain 1990

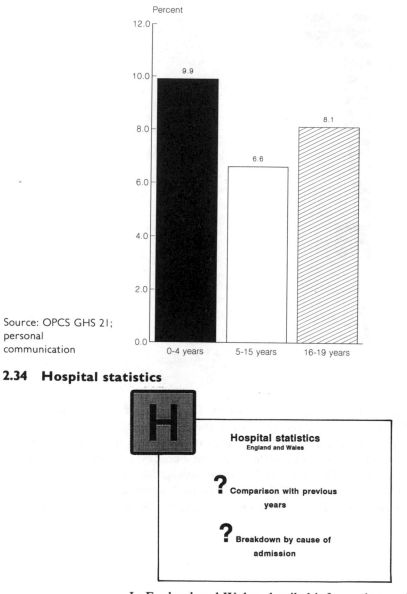

Percent

Source: OPCS GHS 21;
personal
communication

2.34 Hospital statistics

Hospital statistics
England and Wales

? Comparison with previous years

? Breakdown by cause of admission

In England and Wales, detailed information on hospital admissions has not been available by cause since 1985. In 1985 the main cause of hospital admission in childhood (0–14) was respiratory illness (DHSS/OPCS MB4/26). The quality of data collected by new systems, introduced from 1986 onwards as a result of the Körner reports (Steering Group on Health Services Information 1982), is only now becoming adequate for analysis by diagnosis on a national scale. Köner statistics are not directly comparable with data for previous years.

2.35 Causes of hospital admission age 0–4 years, Scotland 1990

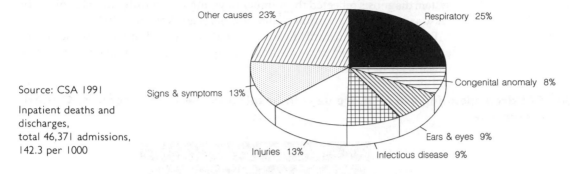

Source: CSA 1991

Inpatient deaths and
discharges,
total 46,371 admissions,
142.3 per 1000

2.36 Causes of hospital admission age 5–14 years, Scotland 1990

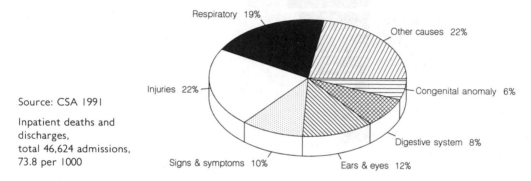

Source: CSA 1991

Inpatient deaths and
discharges,
total 46,624 admissions,
73.8 per 1000

2.37 Causes of hospital admission age 15–24 years, Scotland 1990

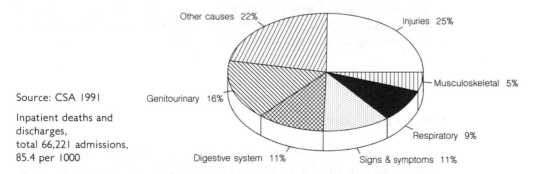

Source: CSA 1991

Inpatient deaths and
discharges,
total 66,221 admissions,
85.4 per 1000

More recent information on hospital admissions by cause is available from
Scotland. The pattern of admissions to Scottish hospitals in 1990 was similar
to that shown in England and Wales in 1985. The largest cause of admission at
0–4 years was a respiratory condition, while at 5–14 injuries were the largest
cause and respiratory problems came next. Among young people aged 15–24

47

the largest cause was injury. The frequency of admissions with a genitourinary system diagnosis reflected the number of young women attending for obstetric reasons, including abortion (Common Services Agency 1991).

Because cause is recorded each time patients are admitted, illnesses which entail repeated short stays in hospital appear more prominent than those which lead to fewer, longer stays.

2.38 Children spending five or more days in hospital in the year: diagnosis, Oxford region 1984

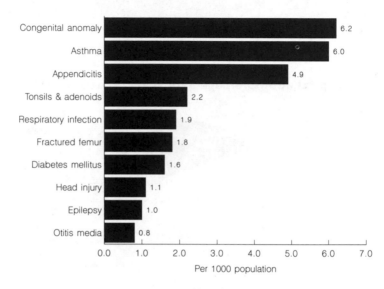

Source: Henderson
et al. 1992

The Oxford Record Linkage Study overcomes some of the limitations of routine hospital statistics by linking together all admissions of the same individual. The principal reasons for children aged 1–14 years being in hospital in 1984, measured by the number of children spending a total of five or more days in hospital at any time in the year, were congenital anomalies, asthma and appendicitis (Henderson *et al.* 1992).

Selected conditions

This section briefly reviews the epidemiology of the principal causes of childhood mortality and morbidity in the UK. Conditions have been selected because they affect a large number of children, there is potential for prevention, they are severe or cause long-term disability, or they attract public interest. Some types of mortality and morbidity are described elsewhere – accidental injuries in Chapter 4, and teenage abortion, drug abuse and the consequences of drunk driving in Chapter 5.

Congenital disorders are an important cause of illness and death in childhood, and contribute to long-term disability. The term 'congenital anomalies' is used here to refer to physical malformations or syndromes present at birth, while 'congenital disorders' includes all conditions which can be inherited.

2.39 Notifications of selected congenital anomalies, England and Wales 1990

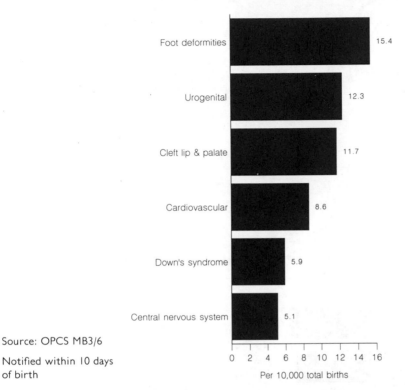

Source: OPCS MB3/6

Notified within 10 days of birth

Per 10,000 total births

The primary purpose of the national reporting system for congenital anomalies, set up in 1964 following the thalidomide epidemic, is to detect rapidly any change in the frequency of a particular condition. Because notifications are limited to conditions identified up to ten days after birth (seven days until 1990) those not always recognized at birth, for example cardiovascular anomalies, are less complete.

In 1990, 1.2 percent of live births in England and Wales were notified with a congenital anomaly. The rate was higher in boys than in girls, most of the difference being due to anomalies of the male genitals. Only serious anomalies are now notified; many of the less serious were excluded from the notification system in 1990, leading to a 36 percent fall in the proportion of total births reported as affected compared to 1989 (OPCS MB3/6).

It is well known that the risk of Down's syndrome increases steeply for mothers over the age of 35. However, most Down's syndrome births are to mothers *under* 35, as younger women have more babies (see Chapter 1).

2.40 Trend in central nervous system anomalies, England and Wales 1979–90

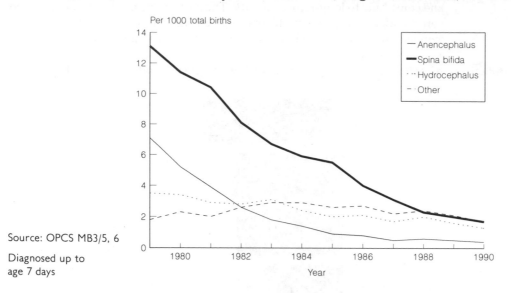

Per 1000 total births

Legend:
— Anencephalus
━ Spina bifida
··· Hydrocephalus
– · Other

Year

Source: OPCS MB3/5, 6

Diagnosed up to
age 7 days

2.41 Stillbirths and infant mortality from congenital anomalies: mother's country of birth, England and Wales 1981–5

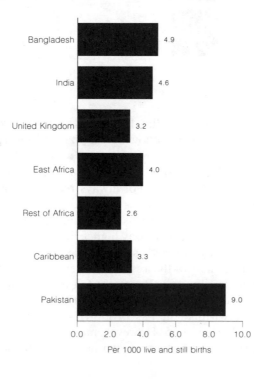

Country	Per 1000 live and still births
Bangladesh	4.9
India	4.6
United Kingdom	3.2
East Africa	4.0
Rest of Africa	2.6
Caribbean	3.3
Pakistan	9.0

Per 1000 live and still births

Source: Balarajan et al.
1989a

50

The rate of serious congenital anomalies reported soon after birth has remained fairly constant for the last decade, with the exception of central nervous system (CNS) anomalies. The long-term decline in CNS anomalies since at least 1969 is continuing and similar decreases have been reported in the Netherlands, Scandinavia, Canada, Hungary and Australia. Although the CNS notification rate fell most sharply for those conditions likely to be detected by neonatal screening, abortion following identification of an affected fetus is not the major explanation for this decline (Baird *et al.* 1991; Chief Medical Officer 1991).

Congenital anomalies are more common in infants of mothers born in Pakistan, causing 33 percent of stillbirths and infant deaths. Mortality in children of Pakistani mothers from limb and musculoskeletal, genitourinary and central nervous system anomalies is particularly high. Risk factors are thought to include high fertility, cultural and religious obstacles to prenatal screening and abortion of affected fetuses, and consanguineous marriages (Bundey *et al.* 1991).

2.42 Likely trends in congenital disorders associated with severe learning disability, England and Wales 1980 and 2000

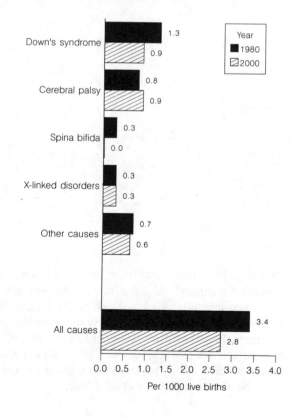

Source: Alberman *et al.* 1992

51

Severe learning disability, defined as having an IQ less than 50, occurred in 3.4 per 1000 live births in England and Wales in the early 1980s, before the introduction of prenatal screening. The main single causes of severe learning disability are Down's syndrome, cerebral palsy, spina bifida and X-linked disorders. Severe learning disability is present in 80 percent of children born with Down's syndrome, 15 percent with spina bifida, 35 percent with cerebral palsy and 75 percent with fragile X syndrome. It is estimated that, where the most sensitive prenatal screening services for Down's syndrome and neural tube defects are provided, this rate could fall to 2.75 per 1000 by the year 2000 (Alberman *et al.* 1992).

2.43 Trend in predicted survival with cystic fibrosis: year of birth, England and Wales 1959–90

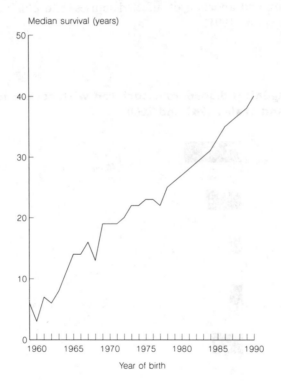

Median survival (years)

Year of birth

Source: Elborn *et al.* 1991

Cystic fibrosis (CF) is the most common of the severe congenital disorders affecting north Europeans. About 1 in 625 couples are both carriers, each child of such a couple having a 1 in 4 risk of the disease (Watson *et al.* 1992). Without screening, which has recently become possible, the prevalence of CF at birth is approximately 0.5 per 1000. However, this may fall if population screening becomes available. Since the 1950s, life expectancy has increased, such that the median life expectancy of a child born in 1990 with CF is estimated to be 40 years (Elborn *et al.* 1992).

Some genetic disorders are especially prevalent in ethnic minority groups. Birth prevalence of sickle cell disease has been estimated as 4 per 1000 Afro-Caribbean births (Royal College of Physicians 1991), but because it is more than twice as common in West African than in Caribbean populations (Horn *et al.* 1986) numbers of affected children cannot accurately be predicted without more precise data on ethnic group. In some inner city districts as many as 2.5 per 1000 of all births may be affected (City and Hackney CHC 1987), making sickle cell disease a major public health issue. In the UK thalassaemia affects an estimated 7 per 1000 Cypriot births, 3.3 per 1000 Pakistani births and 1 per 1000 Indian births (Royal College of Physicians 1991).

2.44 Trend in cerebral palsy: birthweight, Mersey region 1967–84

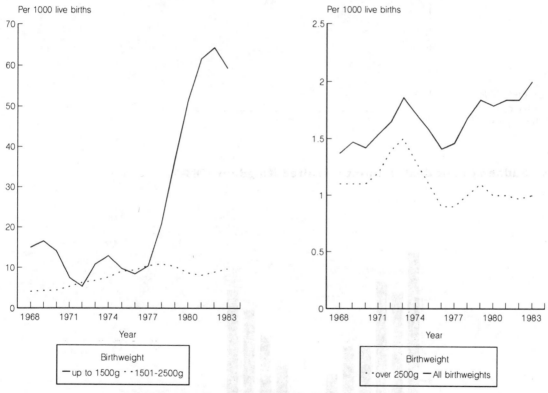

Source: Pharoah *et al.* 1990

Three year averages

Cerebral palsy has increased steeply in the very low weight births (under 1500 g), probably as a result of the increased survival of babies of this weight. On average 9 percent of very low birthweight babies have cerebral palsy (Alberman *et al.* 1992). But as most children born with cerebral palsy weigh over 2500 g and there has been little change in cerebral palsy among heavier babies, the overall rate has remained between 1.5 and 2 per 1000 live births. These data come from a register of infants with cerebral palsy in the Mersey health region in 1967–84 (Pharoah *et al.* 1990).

2.45 Trend in sudden infant death 1980–92, England and Wales, Avon county and Scotland

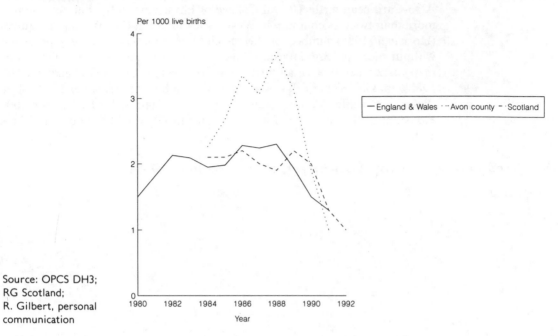

Per 1000 live births

Legend: — England & Wales · · · Avon county - - Scotland

Year

Source: OPCS DH3;
RG Scotland;
R. Gilbert, personal
communication

2.46 Sudden infant deaths: month, United Kingdom 1988–90

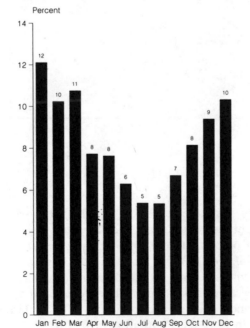

Percent

Jan Feb Mar Apr May Jun Jul Aug Sep Oct Nov Dec

Source: OPCS Monitor
DH3 91/1;
Hansard 1991

Mean 1499 deaths
per year

54

Sudden infant death (SID or 'cot death') is the main cause of postneonatal mortality, making up 44 percent of postneonatal deaths in the UK in 1990. The long-term increase in SID in England and Wales has been reversed since a peak in 1988, falling rapidly to only 456 deaths in 1991–2 (Anonymous 1993). SID occurs most commonly between 1 and 4 months of age, in winter and in boys (OPCS Monitor DH3 91/1; Hansard 1991).

2.47   Postneonatal mortality from sudden infant death: mother's age, England and Wales 1990

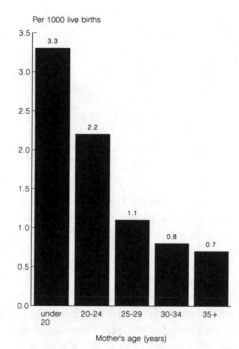

Per 1000 live births

Mother's age (years)

Source: OPCS DH3/24

SID is not a specific diagnosis; the cause of death is, by definition, unknown. Even so, links with younger mothers, low social class and parental smoking are well-established (see Chapters 3 and 4) and it has been suggested that maternal smoking contributes to at least 30 percent of sudden infant deaths (Royal College of Physicians 1992). Recent research has also implicated prone sleeping position, over-wrapping and viral infection (Gilbert *et al*. 1992; Southall and Samuels 1992).

2.48 Trend in mortality age 1–19 years: injuries and other causes, England and Wales 1950–90

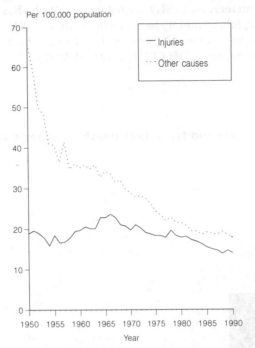

Per 100,000 population

Injuries

Other causes

Year

Source: RG Stat
Review 1930–73;
OPCS DH2

Injuries ICD codes
E800–999

In England and Wales, mortality from injuries at age 1–19 years fell by a quarter over the past 40 years. However, this is a relatively small improvement compared with the decrease in mortality from all other causes taken together, which fell by almost three-quarters in the same period. As a consequence of these trends, injuries are responsible for a growing proportion of all deaths among children and young adults.

This pattern is common to most Western Industrialized countries. It is not clear to what extent advances in treatment leading to the improved survival of injured children have contributed to the downward trend in injury mortality, rather than a fall in the number of injuries, or a decrease in severity. It may be that disability and other long-term effects increased as deaths decreased.

The type of injuries children have and where they occur reflect the age and developmental level of the child. The figure shows childhood mortality from injuries at different stages of development.

Scotland and Northern Ireland have higher mortality than England and Wales at every age except infants. In fact, Scotland and Northern Ireland have rates that are among the worst in Western Europe, whereas England and Wales generally compare favourably (WHO Statistics Annual). Rates for Scotland and Northern Ireland include the small number of deaths under 28 days, whereas those for England and Wales do not.

2.49 Mortality from injuries: age and country, United Kingdom 1987–90

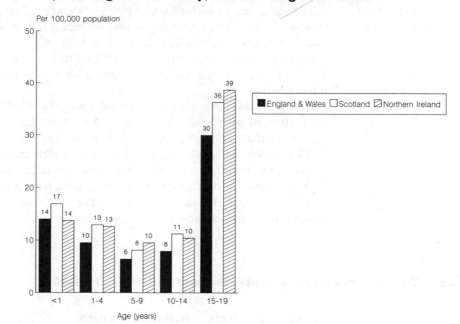

Per 100,000 population

England & Wales ☐ Scotland ☒ Northern Ireland

Age (years)

Source: OPCS DH2;
RG Scotland 1992;
RG N Ireland 1992

2.50 Mortality from injuries: age and sex, England and Wales 1987–90

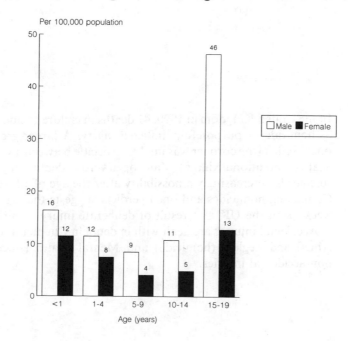

Per 100,000 population

☐ Male ■ Female

Age (years)

Source: OPCS DH2

At all ages, boys have a higher mortality from injuries than girls. The difference increases with age, and by 15–19 years the rate for young men is three-and-a-half times that for young women. Gender differences are also found in hospital admissions. In 1985 in England, one-and-a-half times as many boys under five as girls were admitted to hospital following an injury. For 5–14 year olds, nearly twice as many injured boys were admitted as girls (OPCS MB4/27).

The General Household Survey over the period 1987–9 found that the same proportion of boys under five as girls (5 percent) had an accidental injury needing medical attention in the past three months (OPCS GHS/17–19). The GHS question included attention by a GP, which may be for less serious injuries, and this may account for there being less difference between the sexes than in hospital admissions. For 5–15 year olds, 6 percent of boys compared with 4 percent of girls had such an injury. The difference was greater for young adults (10 percent of men aged 16–24 compared with 4 percent of women).

2.51 Deaths from injuries: cause, England and Wales 1987–90

Age (years)	Accidents %	Homicide %	Suicide %	Open verdict %	Mean deaths per year (100%)
Under 1	71	13	-	16	95
1-4	86	6	-	7	251
5-9	93	3	-	4	202
10-14	90	3	1	7	236
15-19	76	2	12	11	1088
0-19	81	3	7	9	1872
1-19	81	3	7	9	1777

Source: OPCS DH2

In the United Kingdom in 1990, 41 deaths in children under 15 were classified as homicide or purposefully inflicted injury. A larger group were given an open verdict (the coroner was unable to decide between a verdict of accidental death or intentional killing). Many open verdict deaths may be homicide, with suicide also increasingly a possibility after the age of 12 (see Mental health). Combining homicides and open verdicts suggests that up to two children a week die in the UK as a result of deliberate injury – child abuse.

Accidental injuries are dealt with in detail in Chapter 4. In this chapter, see Abuse and neglect (homicide) and Mental health (suicide) for more on non-accidental injuries.

2.52 Child abuse

Reported child abuse is increasing

But its true extent is unknown

Physical and psychological harm resulting from child abuse and neglect are important health problems which are difficult to quantify. Except for the rare cases which result in death and larger numbers which become the subject of a prosecution, little is known about the extent of physical and sexual abuse of children. Proxy measures are provided by the number of children on social services child protection registers and taken into care (see Chapter 3) for these reasons.

Child abuse is closely linked to deprivation, family breakdown and parental stress owing to unemployment and financial problems. Debt was the most common factor mentioned by parents of children registered because of neglect in 1988–90 (NSPCC 1992).

Until the 1980s child sexual abuse was rarely reported in the UK. The surveys that have been carried out are difficult to interpret and its prevalence is not known. The increase in the number of children coming to the attention of health and social services may be because of a true increase in abused children or increased public and professional awareness.

2.53 Homicide and other fatal injuries, infants: cause, England and Wales 1987–90

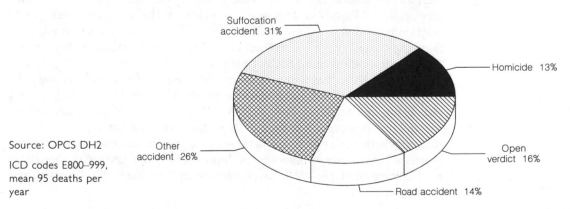

Source: OPCS DH2

ICD codes E800–999, mean 95 deaths per year

Suffocation accident 31%

Homicide 13%

Open verdict 16%

Road accident 14%

Other accident 26%

2.54 Children on child protection registers: age and cause, England 31 March 1992

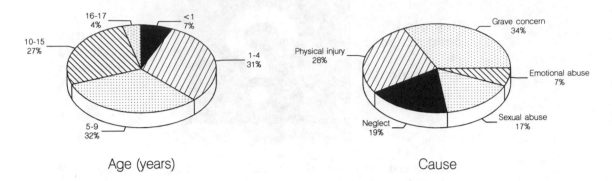

Age (years)   Cause

Source: DH 1993

Total of percentages by cause exceeds 100 because some children are counted in more than one category

National data have been compiled from local authority child protection registers in England since 1989. The number of children on a register at 31 March increased from 41,200 in 1989 to 45,300 in 1991. Changes in registration following the implementation of the Children Act in October 1991 reduced the number to 38,600 in 1992.

Of all children and young people under 18 years of age, 4 per 1000 are included on a register at any one time. Children under 5 years old are the most likely to be included. 'Grave concern', where abuse or neglect is suspected, is the reason for a third of children being on a register. Girls are more likely to be included than boys, the difference occurring at age 10–15, when girls are three times more likely than boys to be on a register because of sexual abuse. Only a minority of the children on registers are looked after by their local authority, the remainder being supported at home by health and social services.

Respiratory disease is a major cause of death, disability and use of health services in childhood (see Morbidity overview), with chest (lower respiratory tract) infections and asthma predominating. Deaths and hospital admissions from chest infections have declined in the last 20 years although they remain the most important numerically (Anderson 1986).

Although there has been concern that deaths from asthma may be increasing in childhood, the evidence suggests this is only for 15–19 year olds (Anderson and Strachan 1991; OPCS DH2). However, hospital admissions for childhood asthma have more than doubled since the mid-1970s. It is unclear whether this reflects an increase in the prevalence or severity of disease (perhaps related to environmental pollution or maternal smoking), changes in medical care, or diagnostic labels (Anderson and Strachan 1991; Strachan and Anderson 1992).

2.55 Trend in deaths from asthma 1974–90: age, England and Wales

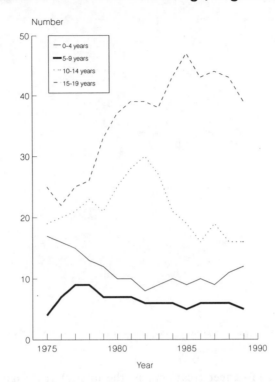

Number

Legend:
- 0-4 years
- 5-9 years
- 10-14 years
- 15-19 years

Year

Source: OPCS DH2

Three year averages

2.56 Cancer registrations age 0–19 years: type, England and Wales 1986

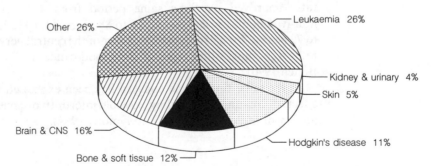

Other 26%

Leukaemia 26%

Kidney & urinary 4%

Skin 5%

Hodgkin's disease 11%

Brain & CNS 16%

Bone & soft tissue 12%

Source: OPCS MB1/19

Total 1482 registrations

In 1986 the national cancer registration system for England and Wales reported 1482 newly diagnosed cases of cancer in children and young people up to 19 years old, a rate of 0.11 per 1000. Fifty-seven percent of cases were boys. Cancer incidence in childhood is most common up to four years old; the lowest incidence is in the 5–9 age group, followed by a steady increase throughout life (OPCS MB1/19). Leukaemia is the most common cancer in younger children, and Hodgkin's disease in adolescence.

2.57 Trend in childhood leukaemia: five-year survival, Great Britain 1971–85

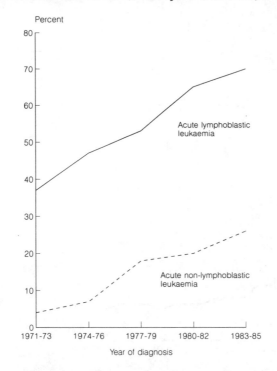

Source: Stiller and
Bunch 1990

Age under 15 years
at diagnosis

Advances in cancer treatment in the last 20 years have greatly increased survival rates. Whereas only 37 percent of children diagnosed with acute lymphoblastic leukaemia in 1971–3 were still alive five years later, for those diagnosed in 1983–5 the proportion was 70 percent. The five-year survival rates improved over the same period from 4 to 26 percent for acute non-lymphoblastic leukaemia, 76 to 88 percent for Hodgkin's disease and 61 to 72 percent for astrocytoma, a cancer of the central nervous system. Survival rates from most other types of childhood cancer also improved (Stiller and Bunch 1990).

At the same time, some concern has been expressed about the long-term effects of treatment, including possible infertility or genetic damage, and the quality of life of survivors (Anonymous 1992).

The common infectious diseases have historically been a major cause of childhood mortality in the UK, and still are in many parts of the world. Measles vaccine was introduced in 1968. Following the new measles, mumps and rubella (MMR) vaccine in 1989, annual measles notifications fell rapidly, and reached an all-time low of less than 10,000 in 1991 (in England and

2.58 Trend in measles notifications 1957–91, England and Wales

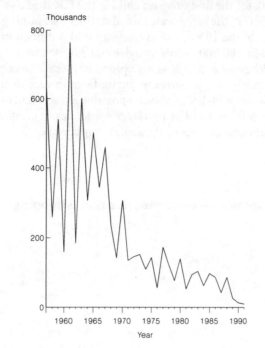

Source: OPCS/PHLS
MB2

2.59 Trend in whooping cough notifications 1957–91, England and Wales

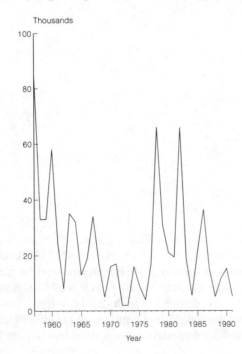

Source: OPCS/PHLS
MB2

Wales). About half of all cases of measles are notified (Clarkson and Fine 1985). In 1990, for the first time, no child in the UK died as a result of measles.

Similarly, before the large scale introduction of whooping cough (pertussis) immunization in the 1950s, the average annual notifications in England and Wales exceeded 100,000, while provisional notifications for 1990 were just over 5000. Whooping cough is an epidemic disease occurring in four-year cycles. Incidence is very sensitive to fluctuations in vaccine uptake, so that the controversy in the mid-1970s about a possible association of vaccination with brain damage was followed by two large epidemics. It is estimated that reports include only about a quarter of the actual number of cases of whooping cough.

2.60 Trend in immunization uptake 1970–89: measles and whooping cough vaccine, England

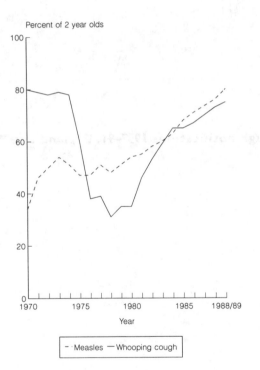

Source: DH Statistical Bulletins 1987–91

While national (England and Wales) uptake of immunization in 1990 was 93 percent for diphtheria, polio and tetanus (DPT) vaccine, 90 percent for measles, mumps and rubella (MMR) vaccine and 88 percent for whooping cough vaccine, some districts had rates as low as 61 percent. These were more deprived, inner city districts which tend to have problems with mobile populations, in some cases large numbers of families in temporary accommodation, and often inadequately resourced primary care services.

Rubella in childhood is not a serious condition, but if contracted by a woman in early pregnancy can lead to death or malformation in the fetus. In 1989, 24,570 cases of rubella were notified in the UK and seven babies were born with congenital rubella (Miller *et al.* 1991).

A national study of tuberculosis in 1978–9 estimated 90 cases per 100,000 Indian and 130 per 100,000 Pakistani and Bangladeshi children aged under 15 in England, compared to 3.6 per 100,000 White children. Rates among UK-born Asian children were about half the rates among those born abroad (MRC TCDU 1982). These rates are probably due to infection acquired abroad, where tuberculosis is more common, transmission from adults born abroad and poor living conditions. Due to concern that tuberculosis may be increasing, a new survey took place in 1992–3.

Of the less common infectious diseases, there are now only one or two cases of diphtheria and polio a year, usually contracted abroad. Meningitis has a relatively high mortality rate and can cause permanent disability. In 1990 there were 1424 notifications and 165 deaths from all types of meningococcal infections in the UK. The commonest cause of viral meningitis is mumps (Isaacs and Menser 1990). Haemophilus influenzae b (Hib) is the commonest cause of bacterial meningitis in children under 5 years. From October 1992, Hib vaccine has been offered at the same time as DTP vaccine.

2.61   HIV-I infection in children aged under 15 years at diagnosis: exposure category, UK cumulative to 31 July 1992

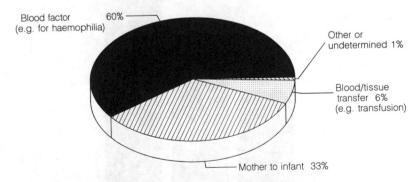

Source: PHLS, personal communication

Total 403 children

From the beginning of the acquired immunodeficiency syndrome (AIDS) epidemic to the end of July 1992, a total of 403 children under 15 years of age in the UK had been diagnosed as infected with human immunodeficiency virus (HIV-1). Forty-seven of these had died. Transmission from mother to baby is increasingly important.

2.62   Trend in prevalence of diabetes at age 10–11 years; 1956, 1968 and 1980, Great Britain

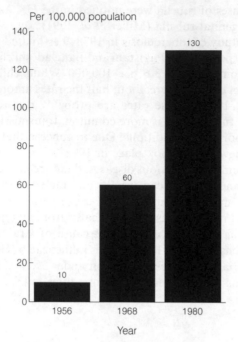

Per 100,000 population

2.63   Incidence of diabetes: age, British Isles 1988

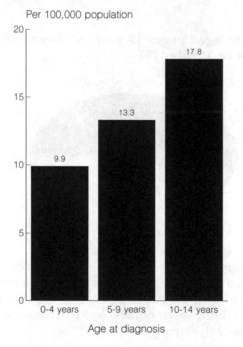

Per 100,000 population

In 1988 it was estimated that there were 19,000 children and teenagers under 20 in the UK with diabetes, with 3200 new cases diagnosed each year (Nabarro 1988). Incidence increases with age, with a peak at 12 years (among children under 15). A survey in 1988 found an incidence of 13.5 per 100,000 children under 15 in the British Isles, varying from 19.8 per 100,000 in Scotland to 6.8 in the Republic of Ireland, after allowing for differences in age composition of the population (Metcalfe and Baum 1991).

The prevalence of childhood diabetes is increasing, as shown by surveys of 10–11 year olds in Britain in 1956, 1968 and 1980. The increase is most marked in higher social classes (Nabarro 1988). Similar trends have been suggested throughout northern Europe (Bingley and Gale 1989).

Mental health problems in children are common, and the OPCS Disability Survey suggests that behaviour problems are the most common cause of functional disability at all ages under 15 (see Morbidity overview).

It is estimated that the prevalence of common psychiatric disorder remains roughly constant throughout childhood although the types of disorder change. A study in an outer London borough in 1982 found 15 percent of three year old children had mild problems, 6 percent moderate and 1 per cent severe (Richman *et al.* 1982). Moderate and severe problems were those involving serious functional incapacity and meriting specialist referral. There were no significant sex differences.

2.64 Common psychiatric disorders in childhood and adolescence

Age 5 years	Age 10 years	Age 15 years
Pre-school adjustment disorders	Conduct and emotional disorders	Depression and anxiety states
Behaviour problems	Hyperkinetic syndrome	Anorexia nervosa

Source: P. Graham, personal communication

Between the age of five and puberty, mental health problems are largely conduct disorders, emotional disorders specific to childhood, and mixed conduct/emotional disorders. Prevalence of these types of disorder combined is 5–10 percent in rural and semi-rural areas and 10–20 percent in inner cities. Boys with conduct disorder outnumber girls by two to one, but at this age there is no sex difference in emotional disorders (Graham 1991). Although these rates are from studies carried out in the 1960s and 1970s there is no reason to believe that rates have changed.

About 2 percent of 5–8 year olds are hyperactive, of whom about half also show conduct disorders (Taylor *et al.* 1991). Depression is found in about 10 percent of 11–16 year old girls (Goodyer and Cooper, unpublished). Disorders of mood (anxiety and depression) are found in 15–20 percent of 15–19 year old girls (E. Monck, personal communication). No comparable estimates exist for boys. Anorexia nervosa occurs in about 1 percent of girls aged 15–18 years in the UK and in about 0.1 percent of boys. There are no UK data for obsessive-compulsive disorder, but the prevalence is about 1 percent in the USA, with an equal sex ratio.

In England in 1989–90 there were 17 hospital admissions for mental illness per 100,000 children under 10 years, 67 per 100,000 aged 10–14 and 176 per 100,000 aged 15–19 (DH HPSSS 1992). Data from previous years show twice as many boys as girls under 10 admitted, slightly more boys at 10–14, but slightly more girls than boys at 15–19 (DH HPSSS 1990).

Many children with a chronic physical condition (such as cerebral palsy or epilepsy), or severe learning difficulty also suffer from psychiatric disorders.

2.65   Trend in suicide age 15–19 years, England and Wales 1975–90

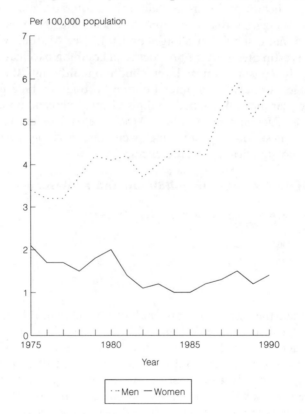

Per 100,000 population

Year

··Men ─Women

Source: OPCS DH2

In England and Wales, the suicide rate for young men aged 15–19 years has climbed steadily since the mid-1970s, whereas the rate for women has remained fairly constant. In 1975, in this age group, twice as many men as women died through suicide; but by 1990 there were over four times as many men. In children aged 12 or less, suicide is rare, with numbers beginning to rise sharply after the age of 14 (OPCS DH2).

2.66 Suicide and other fatal injuries age 15–19 years: cause, England and Wales 1987–90

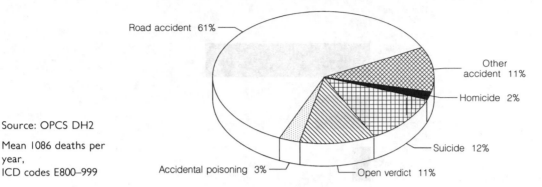

Source: OPCS DH2

Mean 1086 deaths per year,
ICD codes E800–999

Over the period 1987–90 in England and Wales, suicide accounted for 12 percent of injury deaths in the 15–19 age group. A further 11 percent of fatal injuries were given an open verdict. Given the social taboos associated with suicide, there is a reluctance to label a death as such in the face of any degree of uncertainty (Hawton 1986; Sainsbury 1986).

The increase in suicides is thought to be related to social changes over the past two decades, especially increases in the divorce rate and in unemployment (see Chapter 3: Youth unemployment) (Diekstra 1992). At least a quarter of those attempting suicide are diagnosed as having a serious psychiatric disorder (Taylor and Stansfeld 1984).

In contrast to suicide, deliberate self-harm that does not lead to death occurs mainly in young women and has increased since the mid-1960s. It has been estimated that deliberate self-harm is at least 20 times more common than suicide (Brooksbank 1985), which could mean an incidence of up to 2 per 1000 young women. The causes of self-harm are complex, and routine data cannot distinguish between 'failed' suicides and other self-harming behaviour. Episodes of self-harm may be repeated, but rarely lead to death.

Hearing or vision impairment (excluding mild eye defects for which glasses are worn) affects around 3 percent of all children (OPCS GHS). Temporary hearing problems in children, often due to ear infections, are common and rarely of long-term significance. However, children with severe deafness can have their development impaired and suffer behavioural problems. Similarly, most defective eyesight can be corrected with glasses and does not cause any serious handicap. Complete or partial blindness is most often due to inherited conditions.

2.67 Sensorineural deafness: birthweight, children born 1984–8, Oxford Region

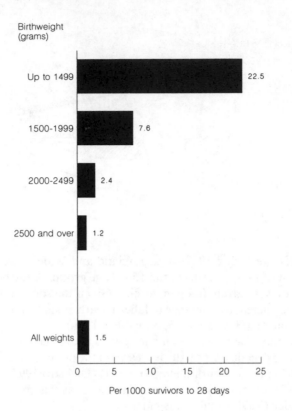

Birthweight
(grams)

Source: Oxford
Register 1991

Per 1000 survivors to 28 days

The most recent national estimate of deafness in children, based on parental reports, was from the OPCS Disability Survey in 1985. This study found that 8 per 1000 children in Great Britain aged 5–9 years and 6 per 1000 aged 10–15 had some level of hearing loss. Severe hearing problems, defined as 'difficulty hearing someone talking in a loud voice in a quiet room' affected 2 per 1000 aged 5–9 and 1 per 1000 aged 10–15 (Bone and Meltzer 1989). In 1977, 92 percent of severe deafness, defined as a hearing loss of 50 dB or more, was sensorineural (nerve deafness). Sixteen percent of sensorineural deafness among eight year olds was caused by congenital rubella (EC Commission 1979). Deafness has almost certainly declined among children following the introduction of rubella vaccine in 1970 for school girls and susceptible women and in 1988 for pre-school children.

For children born in 1984–8, the Oxford Region Register of Early Childhood Impairments reported 1.2 children with sensorineural deafness per 1000 births and 1.5 per 1000 survivors to 28 days. The rate of deafness in survivors to 28 days was 15 times higher in babies weighing under 1500 g at birth than in all babies (Oxford Register 1991).

2.68 Prevalence of defective vision age 10 years: severity, Great Britain 1980

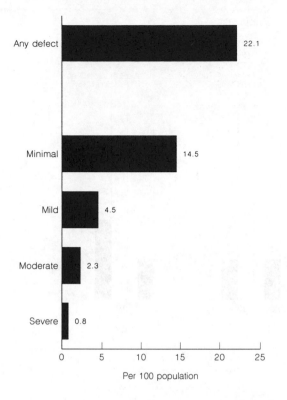

Source: Stewart Brown
and Butler 1985

Visual acuity was tested in children aged 10 in 1980. A mild defect was found in 4.5 percent of children, a moderate defect in 2.3 percent and a severe defect in 0.8 percent (Stewart Brown and Butler 1985). Visual defects are more common in girls than boys and occur more often in children of fathers with non-manual occupations (Peckham 1986).

The OPCS disability survey estimated the prevalence of 'seeing disability' as 2 per 1000 children under 16. The definition included children who could not see well enough to recognize someone they knew across a road (Bone and Meltzer 1989). Data from the Oxford Region Register suggest that some 29 percent of severe vision loss is associated with cerebral palsy.

In England at 31 March 1988, 0.1 per 1000 children under five years old and 0.3 per 1000 aged 5–15 were registered as blind and similar numbers registered as 'partially sighted'. As registration is voluntary, these figures do not reflect the real extent of visual impairment in children. The principal causes of blindness in registered children were disorders of the optic nerve and related parts of the central nervous system; congenital anomalies also played an important part, and were the largest cause of partial sight (DH 1991b).

2.69   Trend in overweight and obese 16–24 year olds, Great Britain 1980 and 1986–7

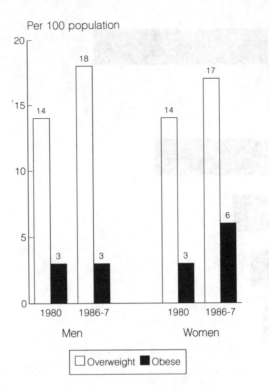

Source: Knight 1984;
Gregory 1990

Being overweight or obese (extremely overweight) contributes to illness in childhood and increases the risk of disease in later life. A trend in the number of schoolchildren who are too heavy for their height has yet to be discerned, but the proportion of young adults appears to have increased. The relationship between weight and height can be summarized by (weight (kg)/height (m))² the body mass index (BMI). Overweight is defined as a BMI of 25–30 and obese as over 30 (Royal College of Physicians 1983). By these definitions 18 percent of young men and 17 percent of young women were overweight in 1986–7, an increase from the previous six years. The proportion of obese young women doubled in this period.

It has been taken as a sign of improved health that height has increased on average during this century. This secular trend was shown in a national survey of 5–11 year olds in England and Scotland for the period 1972–9. The increase was attributed in part to decreasing family size. The trend in increasing height has continued to 1990 (Chinn *et al.* 1989; Chinn and Rona 1993).

Concern about being overweight, and consequent dieting, is common among teenage girls (Wardle and Marsland 1990). Diet and exercise are considered in Chapter 5.

2.70 Five year olds with experience of dental caries: regions, Great Britain 1989–90

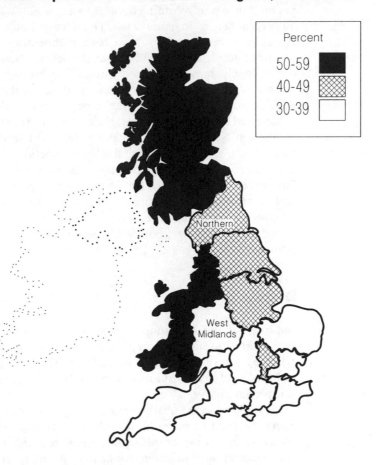

Percent

50-59 ■
40-49 ▨
30-39 □

Northern

West Midlands

Source: Evans and
Dowell 1991

There has been improvement in the last decade in the state of children's dental health, largely owing to fluoride in toothpaste and drinking water, and a reduction in sugar in children's diets (Smith and Jacobson 1988; Downer 1989). However, the number of children with experience of tooth decay remains high. According to the Secretary of State for Health (1991), 'There is no clinical reason why dental decay in children should not virtually be eliminated'.

Dental health is often measured by number of teeth that are decayed, missing or filled (d.m.f.), the caries 'experience'. Five year olds had a mean of 1.8 d.m.f. deciduous teeth at the last decennial UK survey in 1983. The mean number of d.m.f. permanent teeth among 12 year olds was 3.1 (Todd and Dodd 1985). These levels persisted despite declines in the previous 10 years of 50 percent in the proportion of five year olds with caries experience and 40 percent in the proportion of 12 year olds (Downer 1989). The most recent survey indicates that the trend among five year olds is now levelling off (Evans and Dowell 1991).

73

Fluoride is normally present in water at a concentration of about 0.1 parts per million (p.p.m.). Adding fluoride to a concentration of 1 p.p.m. results in a 60 percent decline in dental caries (Faculty of Public Health Medicine 1992). No adverse health effects have been demonstrated. In some parts of the country fluoride occurs naturally at this level. Elsewhere, fluoridation of the water supply may be carried out at the request of the District Health Authority. Fluoridation was first carried out in the 1960s, but it is still not widespread owing largely to public opposition.

Regional comparison of dental health shows a north to south gradient, with children in Northern Ireland having the worst teeth in the UK (Todd and Dodd 1985). Within Great Britain, the proportion of five year olds with caries experience is highest at 59 percent in Scotland and lowest at 31 percent in South West Thames. The Chief Dental Officer, pointing out that the Northern and West Midlands Regions – which have the most extensive fluoridation schemes – have lower caries levels than expected, has recommended that the introduction of new fluoridation schemes should be vigorously pursued (Downer 1989).

Discussion

Improved living conditions, advances in family planning, and increased availability and effectiveness of health care, especially since the creation of the NHS, have resulted in child mortality in the UK today reaching its lowest recorded level (see Mortality overview). However, many childhood deaths are still preventable.

Most (58 percent) deaths before the age of 20 are in the first year of life; many are due to congenital disorders. Screening during pregnancy and the choice of abortion of affected fetuses has the potential to reduce the prevalence at birth of severe congenital disorders. Because of the severe and incurable nature of many congenital disorders, the majority of couples would probably prefer to avoid the birth of an affected child (Royal College of Physicians 1989).

Prematurity and low birthweight are major causes of stillbirths and neonatal mortality. The principal cause of postneonatal mortality is sudden infant death. Postneonatal deaths are strongly associated with parental smoking, both before and after birth (see Chapter 4).

In later childhood and adolescence, injuries – which cause 47 percent of deaths at 1–19 years – stand out as eminently preventable (see Chapter 4). Striking variations by gender and social class emphasize the extent of unnecessary mortality. If mortality from injuries in boys and young men matched that in girls and young women, there would have been on average 850 fewer deaths each year from 1987 to 1990 (age 0–19). Prevention of accidental injuries is discussed further in Chapter 4.

In contrast to the long-term trend in mortality, available measures of morbidity suggest an increase in the prevalence of childhood chronic illness over the last 20 years. This might also reflect changes in perceptions of health and expectations of the availability of health services.

Survival of children with congenital and life-threatening disorders has improved. A child born now with cystic fibrosis can expect to live not only through adolescence but into middle age. Survival of children with cancer has also improved greatly. More premature and low birthweight babies are born alive and live through infancy than in the past, but they may face increased risk of long-term illness.

Respiratory conditions such as asthma, which are the largest element in reported longstanding illness, have shown a steady rise. The reasons for this are not clear, but air pollution such as road traffic emissions may be involved (Chapter 4). Diabetes seems to have become more common, and age of onset may be becoming earlier.

This increase in chronic illness and longer survival of children with severe conditions will have important implications for families and for health service resources.

References

Publications other than routine data series

Alberman, E. *et al.* (1992) *Severe Learning Disability in Young Children: Likely Future Trends*. London, Wolfson Institute of Preventive Medicine.

Anderson, H. R. (1986) 'Respiratory disease in childhood', *British Medical Bulletin* 42: 167–71.

Anderson, H. R. (1989) 'Increase in hospital admissions for childhood asthma: trends in referral, severity and readmissions from 1970 to 1985 in a health region of the United Kingdom', *Thorax* 44: 614–19.

Anderson, H. R. and Strachan, D. P. (1991) 'Asthma mortality in England and Wales, 1979–89', *British Medical Journal* 337: 1357.

Anonymous (1992) 'How can one assess damage caused by treatment of childhood cancer?' (Editorial), *Lancet* 340: 758–9.

Anonymous (1993) 'Headlines', *British Medical Journal* 306: 1562.

Audit Commission (1991) *Measuring Quality: the Patient's View of Day Surgery*. NHS occasional papers no. 3. London, HMSO.

Baird, P. A., Sadovnik, A. D. and Yee I. (1991) 'Maternal age and birth defects: a population study', *Lancet* 337: 527–9.

Bakketeig, L. and Hoffman, H. (1979) 'Perinatal mortality by birth order within cohorts based on sibship size', *British Medical Journal* ii: 693–6.

Balarajan, R., Soni, Raleigh, V. and Botting, B. (1989a) 'Mortality from congenital malformations in England and Wales: variations by mother's country of birth', *Archives of Disease in Childhood* 64: 1457–62.

Balarajan, R., Soni Raleigh, V. and Botting, B. (1989b) 'Sudden infant death syndrome and postneonatal mortality in immigrants in England and Wales', *British Medical Journal* 298: 716–20.

Bingley, P. J. and Gale, E. A. M. (1989) 'Incidence of insulin dependent diabetes in England: a study in the Oxford region 1985–6', *British Medical Journal* 298: 558–60.

Bone, M. and Meltzer, H. (1989) *The Prevalence of Disability among Children*. OPCS Surveys of Disability in Great Britain, report 3. London, HMSO.

Brooksbank, D. J. (1985) 'Suicide and parasuicide in childhood and early adolescence', *British Journal of Psychiatry* 146: 459–63.

Bundey, S., Alam, H., Kaur, A., Mir, S. and Lancashire, R. (1991) 'Why do UK-born Pakistani babies have high perinatal and neonatal mortality rates?', *Paediatric and Perinatal Epidemiology* 5: 101–14.

Burney, P. G., Chinn, S. and Rona, R. J. (1990) 'Has the prevalence of asthma increased in children? Evidence from the national study of health and growth 1973–86', *British Medical Journal* 300: 1306–10.

Butler, N. R. and Golding, J. (1986) *From Birth to Five*. Oxford, Pergamon Press.

Chalmers, I. and Mutch, L. (1981) 'Are current trends in perinatal practice associated with an increase or a decrease in handicapping conditions?', *Lancet* i: 1415.

Chief Medical Officer, Department of Health (1991) *On the State of the Public Health for the Year 1990*. London, HMSO.

Chinn, S. and Rona, R. J. (1993) Trends in weight-for-height and triceps skinfold thickness for English and Scottish children, 1972–1982 and 1982–1990. In press.

Chinn, S., Rona, R. J. and Price, C. E. (1989) 'The secular trend in height of primary school children in England and Scotland 1972–79 and 1979–86', *Annals of Human Biology* 16: 387–95.

City and Hackney Community Health Council (1987) *Sickle Cell Anaemia and Thalassaemia: Report of a Symposium*. London, CHCHC.

Clarkson, J. A. and Fine, P. E. M. (1985) 'The efficiency of measles and pertussis notification in England and Wales', *International Journal of Epidemiology* 14: 153–68.

Common Services Agency (1991) *Hospital Statistics, Scotland 1991*. Edinburgh, SHHD.

Corby, B. (1990) 'Making use of child protection statistics', *Children in Society* 4(3): 304–14.

Department of Education and Science (1992) *Statistics of Education: Schools, January 1991*. London, DES.

Department of Health (1991a) *Welfare of Children and Young People in Hospital*. London, HMSO.

Department of Health (1991b) 'Causes of blindness and partial sight among children aged under 16, newly registered as blind or partially sighted between April 1987 and March 1990', *Statistical Bulletin* 3(5) 91. London, DH.

Department of Health (1993) *Children Act Report 1992*. London, DH.

Diekstra, R. F. W. (1992) 'Suicide and parasuicide: global perspective', in S. A. Montgomery and N. L. M. Goeting (eds) *Current Approaches: Suicide and Attempted Suicide. Risk Factors, Management and Prevention*. Southampton, Duphar Medical Relations.

Downer, M. C. (1989) 'Time trends in dental decay in young children', *Health Trends* 21: 7–9.

Elborn, J. S., Shale, D. J. and Britton, J. R. (1992) 'Cystic fibrosis: current survival and population estimates to the year 2000', *Thorax* 46: 881–5.

European Community Commission (1979) *Childhood Deafness in the European Community*. EUR Report 6413. Luxembourg, EC.

Evans, D. J. and Dowell, T. B. (1991) 'The dental caries experience of 5-year-old children in Great Britain', *Community Dental Health* 8: 185–94.

Faculty of Public Health Medicine Committee on Health Promotion (1992) *Guidelines for Health Promotion No. 30 – Drinking Water*. London, FPHM.

Gilbert, R., Rudd, P., Berry, P. J. *et al.* (1992) 'Combined effect of infection and heavy wrapping on the risk of sudden unexpected infant death', *Archives of Disease in Childhood* 67: 171–7.

Graham, P. (1991) *Child Psychiatry: a Developmental Approach*, 2nd edn. Oxford, Oxford University Press.

Gregory, J., Foster, K., Tyler, H. and Wiseman, M. (1990) *The Dietary and Nutritional Survey of British Adults*. London, HMSO.

Hack, M., DeMonterice, D., Merkatz, I. R., Jones, P. and Fanaroff, A. A. (1981) 'Rehospitalization of the very-low-birthweight infant', *American Journal of Diseases of Children* 135: 263–6.

Hansard, House of Lords (1991) 'Cot deaths', 531, no. 131: cols WA75–8.

Hawton, K. (1986) 'Suicide in adolescence', in A. Roy (ed.) *Suicide*. Baltimore, MD, Williams and Wilkins.

Henderson, J., Goldacre, M. J., Graveney, M. J. and Simmons, H. M. (1989) 'Use of medical record linkage to study readmission rates', *British Medical Journal* 299: 709–13.

Henderson, J., Goldacre, M. J., Fairweather, J. M. and Marcovitch, H. (1992) 'Conditions accounting for substantial time spent in hospital in children aged 1–14 years', *Archives of Disease in Childhood* 67: 83–6.

Hill, A. M. (1989) 'Trends in paediatric medical admissions', *British Medical Journal* 298: 1479–83.

Horn, M. E. C., Dick, M. C., Frost, B., Davis, L. R., Bellingham, A. J., Stroud, C. E. and Studd, J. W. (1986) 'Neonatal screening for sickle cell diseases in Camberwell: results and recommendations of a two year pilot study', *British Medical Journal* 292: 737–40.

Isaacs, D. and Menser, M. (1990) 'Measles, mumps, rubella and varicella', *Lancet* 335: 1384–7.

Knight, I. (1984) *The Heights and Weights of Young Adults in Great Britain*. London, HMSO.

Medical Research Council Tuberculosis and Chest Diseases Unit (1982) 'Tuberculosis in children in a national survey of notifications in England and Wales, 1978–79', *Archives of Disease in Childhood* 57: 734–41.

Metcalfe, M. A. and Baum, J. D. (1991) 'Incidence of insulin dependent diabetes in children aged under 15 years in the British Isles during 1988', *British Medical Journal* 302: 443–7.

Miller, E., Waight, P. A., Vurdien, J. E. *et al.* (1991) 'Rubella surveillance to December 1990: a joint report from the Public Health Laboratory Service and Congenital Rubella Surveillance Programme', *Communicable Disease Reports* 29 March.

Mutch, L., Newdick, M., Lodwick, A. and Chalmers, I. (1986) 'Secular changes in rehospitalization of very low birth weight infants', *Paediatrics* 78: 164–71.

Nabarro, J. D. N. (1988) 'Diabetes in the UK: some facts and figures', *Diabetic Medicine* 5: 816–22.

National Society for the Prevention of Cruelty to Children (1992) *Child Abuse Trends in England and Wales 1988–90*. London, NSPCC.

Oxford Register of Early Childhood Impairments (1991) *Annual Report*. Oxford, ORECI.

Peckham, C. S. (1986) 'Vision in childhood', *British Medical Bulletin* 42(2): 150–4.

Pharoah, P., Cooke, T., Cooke, R. and Rosenbloom, L. (1990) 'Birthweight-specific trends in cerebral palsy', *Archives of Disease in Childhood* 65: 602–6.

Power, C. (1992) 'A review of child health in the 1958 birth cohort: National Child Development Study', *Paediatric and Perinatal Epidemiology* 6: 81–110.

Richman, N., Stevenson, J. and Graham, P. (1982) *Pre-school to School: a Behavioural Study*. London, Academic Press.

Royal College of Physicians (1983) 'Obesity', *Journal of the Royal College of Physicians* 17: 1.

Royal College of Physicians (1989) *Prenatal Diagnosis and Genetic Screening: Community and Service Implications*. London, RCP.

Royal College of Physicians (1991) *Purchasers' Guidelines to Genetic Services in the NHS*. London, RCP.

Royal College of Physicians (1992) *Smoking and the Young*. London, RCP.

Sainsbury, P. (1986) 'The epidemiology of suicide', in A. Roy (ed.) *Suicide*. Baltimore, MD, Williams and Wilkins.

Secretary of State for Health (1991) *The Health of the Nation*. London, HMSO.

Shaw, C. (1988) 'Components of growth in the ethnic population', *Population Trends* 52: 26–30.

Smith, A. and Jacobson, B. (1988) *The Nation's Health: a Strategy for the 1990s*. London, King's Fund.

Southall, D. P. and Samuels, M. R. (1992) 'Reducing risks in the sudden infant death syndrome' (Editorial), *British Medical Journal* 304: 265–6.

Steering Group on Health Services Information (Körner Committee) (1982) *First Report to the Secretary of State: a Report on the Collection and Use of Information about Hospital Clinical Activity in the NHS*. London, HMSO.

Stewart Brown, S. and Butler, N. (1985) 'Visual acuity in a national sample of 10-year old children', *Journal of Epidemiology and Community Health* 39: 107–12.

Stiller, C. A. and Bunch, K. J. (1990) 'Trends in survival for childhood cancer in Britain diagnosed 1971–85', *British Journal of Cancer* 62: 806–15.

Strachan, D. P. and Anderson, H. R. (1992) 'Trends in hospital admission for asthma in children', *British Medical Journal* 304: 819–20.

Taylor, E., Sandberg, S., Thorley, G. and Giles, S. (1991) *The Epidemiology of Childhood Activity*. Maudsley Monograph 33. Oxford, Oxford University Press.

Taylor, E. A., and Stansfield, S. A. (1984) 'Children who poison themselves. I: A clinical comparison with psychiatric controls', *British Journal of Psychiatry* 145: 127–35.

Thornes, R. (1990) *Just for the Day*. London, Caring for Children in the Health Service.

Todd, J. and Dodd, T. (1985) *Children's Dental Health in the UK 1983*. London, HMSO.

Wadsworth, M. (1987) 'Follow-up of the first national birth cohort: findings from the Medical Research Council National Survey of Health and Development', *Paediatric and Perinatal Epidemiology* 1: 95–117.

Wardle, J. and Marsland, L. (1990) 'Adolescent concerns about weight and eating; a social developmental perspective', *Journal of Psychosomatic Research* 34: 377–91.

Watson, E. K., Mayall, E. S., Lamb, J., Chapple, J. and Williamson, R. (1992) 'Psychological and social consequences of community carrier screening for cystic fibrosis', *Lancet* 340: 217–20.

Welsh Office (1991) *Child Protection Registers: Statistics for Wales 1990*. Cardiff, Welsh Office.

World Health Organisation (1992) *Health for All Indicators Eurostat/PC*. Copenhagen, WHO Regional Office for Europe.

World Population Data Sheet (1992) London, Population Concern.

Routine data series

Office of Population Censuses and Surveys:
  OPCS DH1 Mortality statistics: surveillance (time-trends)
  OPCS DH2 Mortality statistics: cause
  OPCS DH3 Mortality statistics: perinatal and infant
  OPCS DH6 Mortality statistics: childhood
  OPCS FM1 Birth statistics
  OPCS GHS General Household Survey
  OPCS MB1 Cancer statistics: registrations
  OPCS PHLS MB2 Communicable diseases
  OPCS MB3 Congenital malformation statistics
  OPCS MB4 Hospital in-patient enquiry
  OPCS MB5 Morbidity statistics from general practice
  OPCS Monitors are periodic bulletins between the main volumes.
Central Statistical Office:
  CSO Annual Abstract of Statistics (AAS)
Department of Health:
  Health and Personal Social Services Statistics for England (HPSSS)
Registrar General for Northern Ireland:
  RG N Ireland Annual Reports
Registrar General for Scotland:
  RG Scotland Annual Reports

CHAPTER 3

Socioeconomic environment

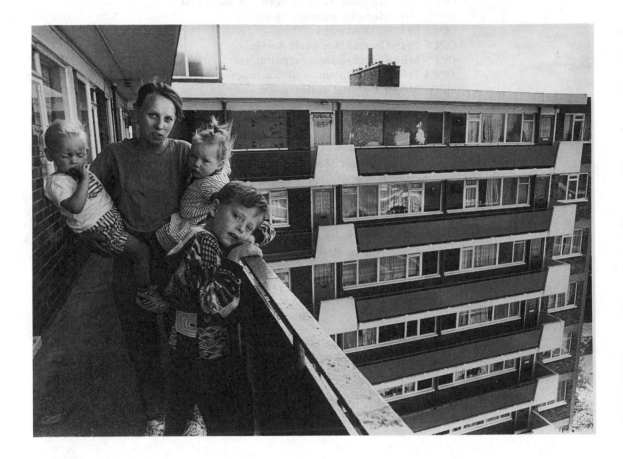

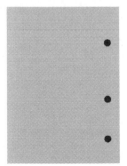

Key facts

- A child in the lowest (unskilled manual) social class is twice as likely to die before age 15 years as a child in the highest (professional) social class (England and Wales 1981 and 1990).

- Other measures of ill-health also show that children in the manual social classes are at a disadvantage.

- An estimated quarter of all children live in poverty, most (54 percent) because of parents' unemployment (Great Britain 1987).

- Four-fifths of children in households whose 'head' is unemployed are in poverty (Great Britain 1987).

- Infant mortality is twice as high for births outside marriage and registered by the mother alone as for births within marriage (England and Wales 1990).

- A higher proportion of children are in poverty in Northern Ireland than elsewhere, followed by the North of England and Wales (1985).

- Areas of socioeconomic deprivation have higher mortality. Inner city Central Birmingham has an infant mortality about three times that in rural Huntingdon (1988–90).

- Some 200,000 children are homeless (Great Britain 1990).

Introduction

It has long been recognized that the socioeconomic environment exerts a powerful influence on health. If all children under 16 had the same chances of survival as the children of doctors, lawyers and managers, child mortality would fall by about a quarter (based on OPCS DS 8, DH3/24). At the end of the twentieth century, despite improvements in the health of the population as a whole, striking inequalities persist (DHSS 1980; Whitehead 1988; Davey Smith *et al.* 1990). This chapter describes the socioeconomic circumstances of British children and some of the consequences for their health.

Children inherit their social position, and as dependents they do not control their own environment, especially during the early years. Comparisons of children living in different circumstances are usually based on the family, often the 'head' of the family. Possibly the most useful measure for such comparison would be income, but suitable data are not generally available. The most common and longest-serving measure of social position is a scale of occupations – the Registrar General's social classes. Information on occupation is relatively easy to collect and is associated with income, income security, education and working conditions.

Inevitably, there are limitations to any single socioeconomic measure. The classification system is historically based on men's full-time employment and is difficult to apply meaningfully to women's occupations, which cluster in the lower non-manual class. A substantial proportion of the population, such as the unemployed, chronically sick and lone parent families with no paid work, are excluded from occupational social class. Because of such inadequacies, alternative classifications using housing ownership and amenities, income and employment status are sometimes used. However, social class provides a useful summary measure and for this reason is still used extensively in national statistics.

A child's social class is taken from the occupation of the 'head of household', usually the father. The social classes are:

Social class		Examples
I	Professional	Doctor, lawyer
II	Managerial	Manager, teacher
IIIN	Skilled non-manual	Clerk, shop assistant
IIIM	Skilled manual	Miner, bricklayer
IV	Partly skilled	Bus conductor, postman
V	Unskilled	Labourer, porter
Other		Armed forces, unoccupied and inadequately described

The contents of this chapter are divided into four sections. The first three deal with health differences between social classes, causes and effects of child poverty, and homeless families. The fourth section briefly describes one of the most disadvantaged groups of children and young people, those in care.

This chapter does not present data on child health in ethnic minorities. Relatively little is known about ethnic differences in children's health in the UK, but ethnic group was included in the Census for the first time in 1991, and will be available in NHS statistics from 1993–4. The particular health situation of ethnic minorities reflects a combination of factors – genetic, socioeconomic and cultural – and these are referred to in Chapter 2 (infant mortality, genetic disorders, infectious disease) and Chapter 5 (diet). To a great extent mortality and morbidity in ethnic minority adults reflect the adverse circumstances which they share with other disadvantaged sections of society, to which may be added the stress of migration and of racism, and language and other barriers to access to services.

Social class

3.1 Social class of live births within marriage, England and Wales 1990

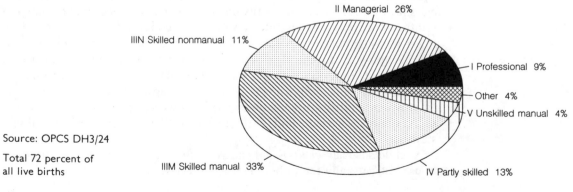

II Managerial 26%

IIIN Skilled nonmanual 11%

I Professional 9%

Other 4%

V Unskilled manual 4%

IIIM Skilled manual 33%

IV Partly skilled 13%

Source: OPCS DH3/24

Total 72 percent of all live births

82

3.2 Social class of children age 1–14 years, Great Britain 1981

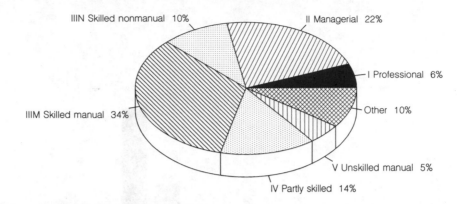

IIIN Skilled nonmanual 10%

II Managerial 22%

I Professional 6%

Other 10%

IIIM Skilled manual 34%

V Unskilled manual 5%

IV Partly skilled 14%

Source: OPCS DS 8

From 1981 Census

Social class is recorded for the 92 percent of births that are within marriage or registered by both parents (OPCS FM1). However, the figure shows the social class of the 72 percent of births within marriage only, as most analyses are available only for these births. Unmarried fathers who register their child's birth have a lower social class distribution than married fathers. Births outside marriage and those where social class is recorded as 'other' consistently show mortality rates similar to social class V.

3.3 Neonatal mortality: social class, England and Wales 1990

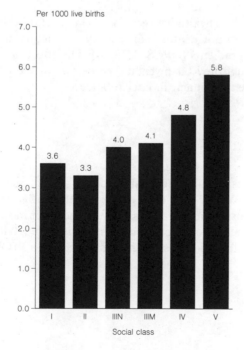

Per 1000 live births

Social class

Source: OPCS DH3/24

Within marriage only

83

3.4   Postneonatal mortality: social class, England and Wales 1990

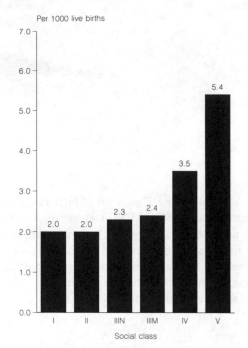

Per 1000 live births

Source: OPCS DH3/24

Within marriage only

Inequalities in child health between social classes start at birth or even earlier. Stillbirths and infant deaths, particularly postneonatal deaths, show pronounced class gradients (OPCS DH3/24). The effect of social class is partly mediated through low birthweight (see below) in the perinatal period and through poor environment in later infancy.

The main causes of infant death show clear social class gradients. In 1990 in England and Wales, the rate of neonatal deaths from non-infectious respiratory disorders in social class V was twice that in social class I. Sudden infant death, the principal cause of postneonatal mortality, was three times more common in social class V than in social class I (OPCS DH3/24).

3.5 Neonatal mortality from respiratory disorder: social class, England and Wales 1990

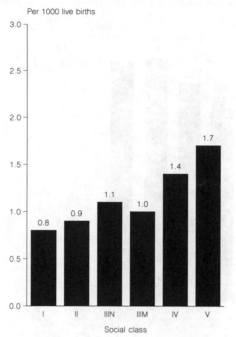

Per 1000 live births

Social class

Source: OPCS DH3/24

Within marriage only

3.6 Postneonatal mortality from sudden infant death: social class, England and Wales 1990

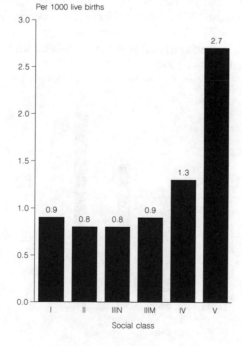

Per 1000 live births

Social class

Source: OPCS DH3/24

Within marriage only

3.7 Low birthweight: social class, England and Wales 1990

Source: OPCS DH3/24

Births under 2500 g, within marriage only

Per 1000 live births

```
80 ┐
   │
70 ┤                              69   68
   │
60 ┤                    62
   │              58
   │         52
50 ┤    47
   │
40 ┤
   │
30 ┤
   │
20 ┤
   │
10 ┤
   │
 0 ┴──I────II───IIIN──IIIM───IV────V──
              Social class
```

The proportion of babies weighing less than 2500 g at birth was 68 per 1000 live births in social class V compared to 47 in class I in 1990 (OPCS DH3/24). Low birthweight is associated not only with greater risk of death in infancy, but also with increased risk of impairments such as cerebral palsy (Chapter 2).

3.8 Infant mortality: social class, standardized for birthweight and maternal age and birth order, England and Wales 1990

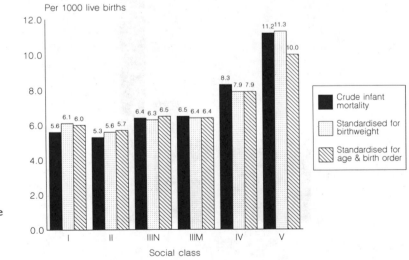

Per 1000 live births

Source: Based on OPCS DH3/24

Births within marriage directly standardized on live births, social classes I to V

Legend:
- Crude infant mortality
- Standardised for birthweight
- Standardised for age & birth order

Values:
- I: 5.6, 6.1, 6.0
- II: 5.3, 5.6, 5.7
- IIIN: 6.4, 6.3, 6.5
- IIIM: 6.5, 6.4, 6.4
- IV: 8.3, 7.9, 7.9
- V: 11.2, 11.3, 10.0

Class differences in infant mortality which might be due to birthweight, mother's age or birth order can be allowed for by standardization. The class gradient in infant mortality is little affected by standardization for birthweight, indicating that the higher mortality in lower social classes is not accounted for by the greater proportion of low birthweight babies in those classes. There is some reduction in the gradient when infant mortality is standardized for mother's age and parity, suggesting that up to a third of the difference between classes I and V is due to the concentration of younger mothers in the lower social classes (based on OPCS DH3/24).

3.9 Mortality (all causes) age 1–14 years: social class, England and Wales 1979–80 and 1982–3

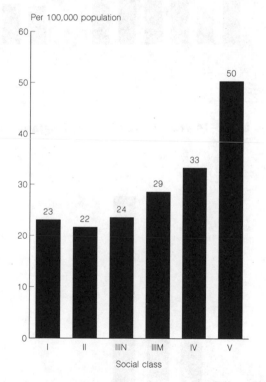

Source: OPCS DS 8

Four year averages

Child mortality shows a gradient by social class at all ages. The advantage for children in higher social classes is evident at each stage of childhood, but is especially pronounced among 1–4 year olds (OPCS DS 8). The most recently published rates are for 1979–83, using deaths data for England and Wales in conjunction with the 1981 Census. The 1991 Census data will be used to provide more up-to-date rates, but these are not yet available.

87

3.10 Mortality (all causes) age 1–14 years: age and social class, England and Wales 1979–80 and 1982–3

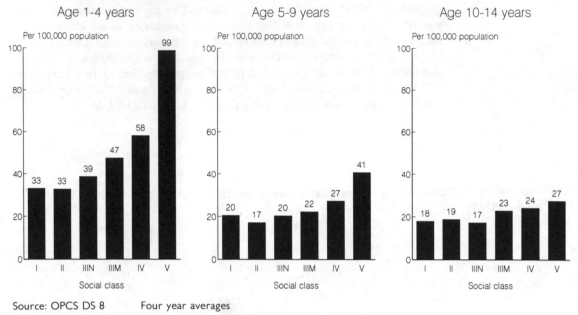

Age 1-4 years   Age 5-9 years   Age 10-14 years

Source: OPCS DS 8   Four year averages

3.11 Mortality from injuries age 1–14 years: social class, England and Wales 1979–80 and 1982–3

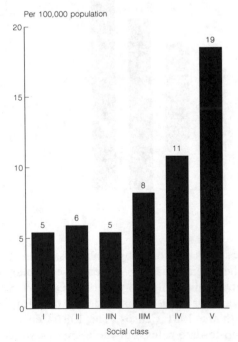

Source: OPCS DS 8

Four year averages

The social class gradient for deaths due to injuries is steeper than for any other cause of child death, a fact that is all the more disturbing since these account for around a third of all deaths of children. Children aged 1–14 years from social class V have a death rate from injuries nearly four times that occurring in class I (OPCS DS 8). There is evidence that non-fatal injuries may also be related to social class in the same way.

3.12 Mortality from traffic collision with pedestrian age 1–14 years: social class, England and Wales 1979–80 and 1982–3

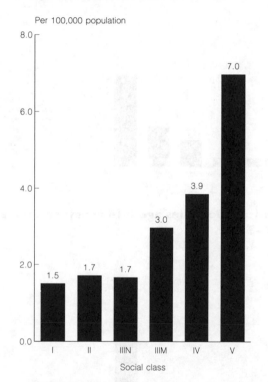

Per 100,000 population

Source: OPCS DS 8

Four year averages

Some types of injuries have particularly steep social class gradients. In the case of road accidents, the major cause of fatal injury in children, the markedly higher risk to children in classes IV and V is probably linked to a greater likelihood of their being on the streets; their families are less likely to own a car and they are less likely to have access to alternative places to play.

Fires are the most common cause of accidental death at home. Children from the manual social classes are at the greatest risk of being the victim of a fire. This is likely to be associated with living in poorer quality housing, possibly without central heating and therefore using less safe heating appliances. Such families may also lack money to buy the safest furnishings and appliances. Only 64 percent of social class V households had central heating, compared to 94 percent in social class I, in 1989 (OPCS GHS 20).

3.13 Mortality from fires age 1–14 years: social class, England and Wales 1979–80 and 1982–3

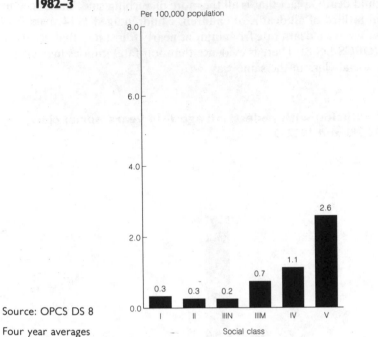

Per 100,000 population

8.0

6.0

4.0

2.0

0.0

2.6
1.1
0.7
0.3   0.3   0.2

I   II   IIIN   IIIM   IV   V

Social class

Source: OPCS DS 8

Four year averages

3.14 Mortality from congenital anomalies age 1–14 years: social class, England and Wales 1979–80 and 1982–3

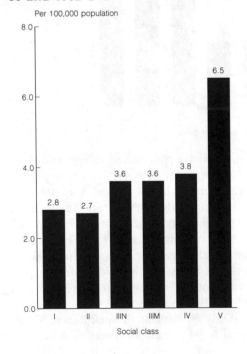

Per 100,000 population

8.0

6.0

4.0

2.0

0.0

6.5
2.8   2.7   3.6   3.6   3.8

I   II   IIIN   IIIM   IV   V

Social class

Source: OPCS DS 8

Four year averages

3.15   Mortality from respiratory conditions age 1–14 years: social class, England and Wales 1979–80 and 1982–3

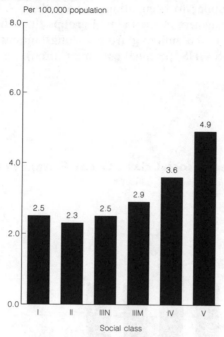

Per 100,000 population

Source: OPCS DS 8

Four year averages

Class gradients are not present for all causes of death, but there is no main cause for which children in lower classes have relatively low rates. Deaths from several major causes of death – infectious diseases, diseases of the respiratory system such as pneumonia, congenital anomalies (particularly anencephaly and spina bifida) – are more common in children from lower social classes (OPCS DS 8).

3.16   Chronic illness age 0–19 years: socioeconomic group (limiting longstanding illness), Great Britain 1991

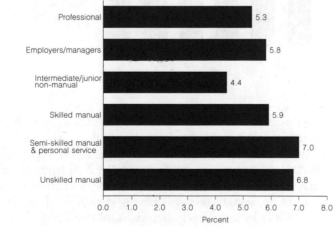

Source: OPCS GHS, personal communication

91

Social class differences can be seen in morbidity statistics as well as in those for mortality. Data from the GHS are analysed by socioeconomic group, a classification similar to occupational social class. A higher proportion of children and teenagers in the manual groups than the non-manual groups were reported to be suffering from a longstanding illness limiting their activities (OPCS GHS, personal communication).

3.17   Regular coughing age 10 years: social class, Great Britain 1980

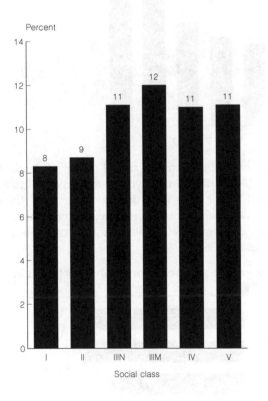

Source: 1970 birth
cohort, unpublished

Data from a national survey of 10 year olds in 1980 show class gradients in symptoms of ill-health. More children in the lower social classes were reported by parents as usually coughing during the day or night than in classes I and II (1970 birth cohort, unpublished). Earlier data from the same study showed a class gradient in serious respiratory illness, with more than twice as many children in social class V than in classes I, II or IIIN having suffered pneumonia by age five (Butler and Golding 1986).

3.18   Pneumonia by age five years: social class, Great Britain 1975

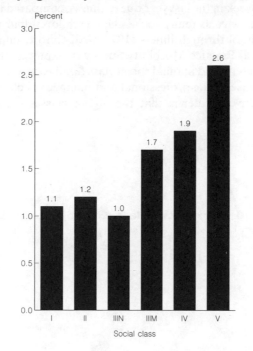

Source: Butler and
Golding 1986

3.19   School absence due to ill-health age 10 years: social class, Great Britain 1980

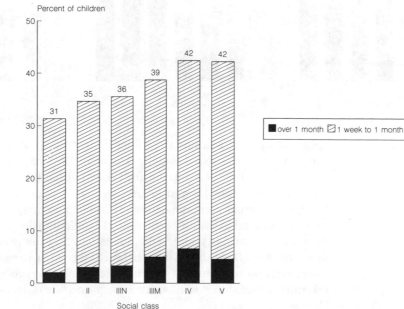

Source: 1970 birth
cohort, unpublished

Absence of one week
or more in the past
year

93

In 1980, 42 percent of social class V children had been absent from school for more than a week in the last year due to illness, compared to 31 percent in class I. More than twice as many social class V children had missed more than a month of school through illness (1970 birth cohort, unpublished).

The General Practice Morbidity Survey (Chapter 2) showed that children from intermediate and manual social class families saw a doctor slightly more often than those in the professional and managerial classes (OPCS MB5/2), although there is evidence that the higher classes consult a doctor more readily.

3.20 Behaviour problems age 10 years: social class, Great Britain 1980

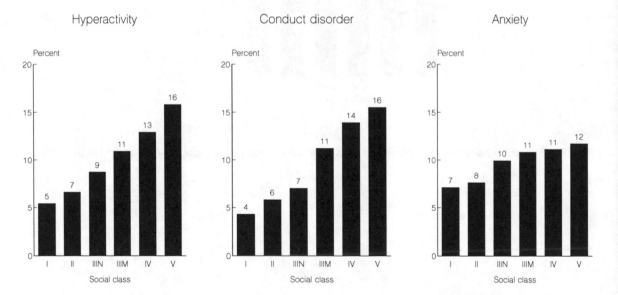

Source: A. Osborn, personal communication

Behavioural and emotional problems are more commonly reported in children with lower social class backgrounds. In a national survey of 10 year olds the percentage of children with behavioural difficulties such as hyperactivity, conduct disorder and anxiety increased with decreasing social class (Osborn, personal communication, 1970 birth cohort).

Measures used to identify behavioural problems in large surveys of children do not equate with psychiatric diagnoses, but they are generally indicative of such problems. Data shown here pertain to the worst 10 percent of children on a behavioural continuum; overall prevalence is predetermined by this arbitrary choice, but it is adequate to demonstrate differences between social classes.

Poverty

3.21 Trend in children and whole population in poverty (living in households below half average income), Great Britain 1979–87

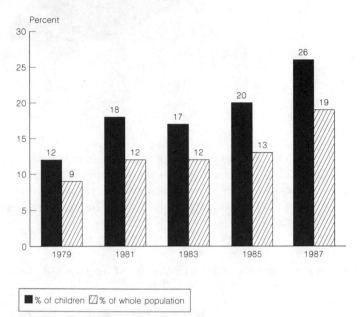

Source: Oppenheim 1990

There is no official definition of poverty in Britain, but the European Community defines half the national mean household income (adjusted for household size and age of children) as the relative poverty line. In 1990 this was £134 a week for a family of two parents and two children (Oppenheim 1990). By this definition, over three million children were living in poverty in Great Britain in 1987.

Between 1979 and 1987 the number of people in poverty in Great Britain more than doubled, from five to ten million. The national average household income rose by 23 percent in real terms, but only by 0.1 percent for the poorest tenth (Oppenheim 1990).

Households that include children are at higher risk of poverty than those that do not. The proportion of children living in poverty was higher than the proportion of the whole population in poverty throughout the 1980s. In 1987, more than a quarter of all children were in households living below the poverty line, compared with less than one-fifth of the population as a whole (DSS 1990).

3.22 Children in poverty: economic status of 'head' of household, Great Britain 1987

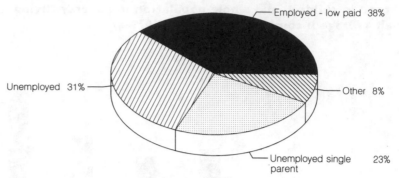

Source: DSS 1990

Total 3 million children

Most of these children (54 percent) are in poverty because of unemployment, including 23 percent where the unemployed 'head of household' is a lone parent. A further 38 percent are in poverty because the 'head of household' is in low paid employment (DSS 1990). The trend in unemployment is shown in Chapter 1.

3.23 Risk of poverty: economic status of 'head' of household, Great Britain 1987

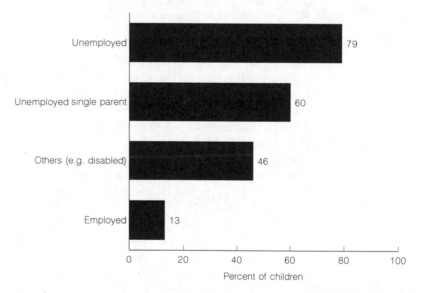

Source: DSS 1990

More than three-quarters of all children in two parent families where the 'head' of household was unemployed and 60 percent of all those with a lone unemployed parent were in poverty, compared with 13 percent of children in two parent families whose heads were in employment (DSS 1990). Because statistics are based on private households, these figures exclude children in homeless families.

3.24   Activities of 16 year olds a year after reaching school-leaving age, Great Britain 1975–88

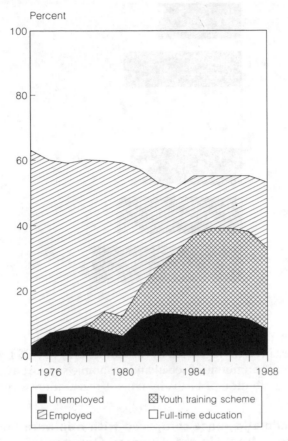

Source: Roll 1990

Unemployment does not only affect children through their parents. Between 1975 and 1988 the proportion of 17 year olds in employment fell by two-thirds. In addition to general economic trends, young people's employment has been affected by the collapse of the apprenticeship system. In 1988, 20 percent of children who had reached school-leaving age went into employment, 8 percent were registered unemployed, 25 percent were on government training schemes and the remainder continued in education (Roll 1990). The true extent of youth unemployment is masked by government training schemes introduced in 1981 and by changes over time in social security regulations.

The number of unemployed 16 and 17 year olds in Great Britain increased from 58,000 in April 1990 to 99,000 in April 1992 (*Employment Gazette* October 1992).

3.25   Infant mortality: registration of birth, England and Wales 1990

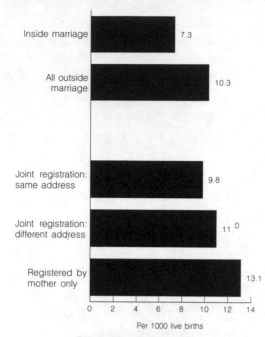

Source: OPCS DH3/24

Per 1000 live births

Infant mortality is higher in births outside marriage than within marriage, and highest in births registered by the mother only (OPCS DH3/24). This gradient reflects the amount of social and economic support available to the mother. The distribution of births by type of registration is shown in Chapter 1.

3.26   Income Support child allowance compared with minimum and average weekly costs of bringing up a child, United Kingdom October 1991

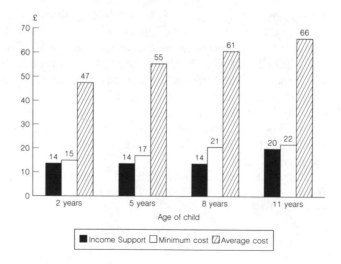

Source: National
Children's Home 1992

98

The means-tested social security benefits on which the poorest families depend are barely adequate compared to the costs of bringing up a child. Income Support child allowance is added to allowances for other needs to make up the household's 'applicable amount'; the benefit paid is only the amount needed to 'top up' the claimant's income to that amount. The child allowance in October 1991 was £13.60 a week for a child up to 10 years old and £20 a week for 11 years and over; at every age this was less than the estimated minimum cost of a child's food, clothing and other needs and less than a third of the average expenditure on a child (outside London) (National Children's Home 1992).

Lone mothers under 18 receive lower rates of income support, both during pregnancy and after birth, than older lone mothers.

3.27 Trend in Child Benefit as percentage of average male manual earnings, Great Britain 1950–90

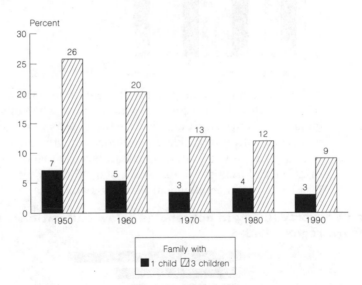

Source: DSS 1991

Child Benefit is payable for all dependent children irrespective of household income, and is usually paid to the mother. In April 1992 Child Benefit was £9.65 a week for the first child and £7.80 a week for each subsequent child. Child Benefit was frozen between 1987 and 1991, and to equal the 1985 level, adjusted for inflation, would now be £10.40 per child. The value of Child Benefit has fallen considerably relative to earnings; in 1950 Child Benefit (then Child Support) for a one child family was worth 7 percent of average male manual earnings, while by 1990 its value had more than halved to 3 percent. For a three child family, the fall was from 26 to 9 percent of male manual earnings (DSS 1991).

3.28 Resources of families with disabled children and all families with children, Great Britain 1985

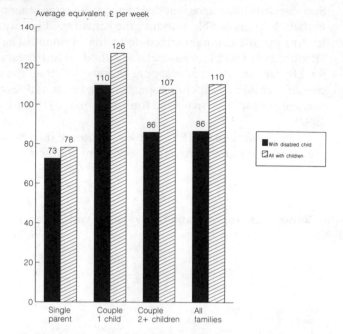

Average equivalent £ per week

■ With disabled child
▧ All with children

Source: Smyth and
Robus 1989

Taking account of both income (benefits plus earnings) and expenditure, families with a disabled child have less resources than other families. Disabled children, as well as their families, are therefore exposed to additional burdens associated with poorer living conditions (Smyth and Robus 1989).

Enquiries into the educational achievement and transition to work of disabled children show that they start their adult lives with additional disadvantages in employment (Walker 1982).

3.29 Children in poverty (living in households below half national average income), UK standard regions 1983–5

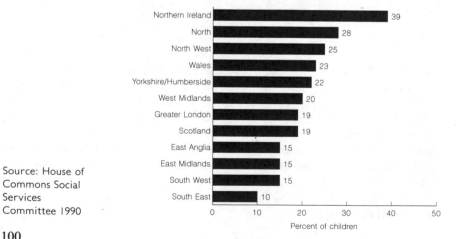

Percent of children

Source: House of
Commons Social
Services
Committee 1990

100

Some parts of the UK are much poorer than others. In 1983–5 the proportion of children who lived in households in poverty (below half of the national average household income) in the most deprived region, Northern Ireland, was, at 39 percent, nearly four times that in South East England excluding Greater London. Wales and the North of England had higher rates of poverty than the South (House of Commons Social Services Committee 1990).

3.30 Infant mortality: regions, United Kingdom 1988–90

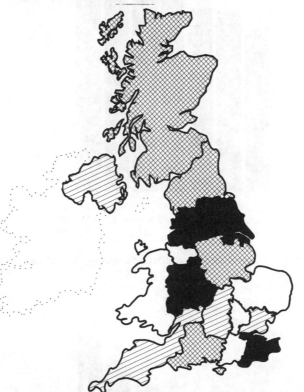

Per 1000 live births	
8.5–10.0	■
7.9–8.4	▨
7.7–7.8	▨
6.7–7.6	□

Source: OPCS Monitor
DH3 91/2;
RG Scotland 1990;
RG N Ireland 1990,
1991

Infant mortality consistently shows large geographical variations within the UK, although a long-term aim of the NHS has been to reduce inequalities in health (DHSS 1976). These geographical differences to a great extent reflect socioeconomic inequality, although the size of the units (standard regions or health regions) obscures the great variation within regions. In 1988–90 infant mortality was 7.9 per 1000 live births in England and Wales, 8.2 in Scotland and 7.8 in Northern Ireland (a three year average is used because of small numbers in a single year).

Higher mortality is generally associated with northern, inner city and economically depressed areas. The lowest 1988–90 infant mortality rate among the Health Districts in England and Wales was 4.7 in rural Huntingdon and the highest was 14.0 in Central Birmingham (OPCS Monitor DH3 91/2).

101

3.31 Infant mortality: area deprivation category, Scotland 1980–2

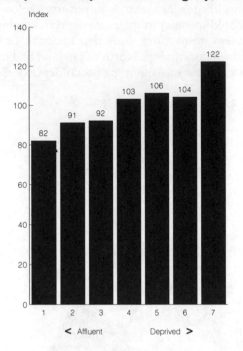

Source: Carstairs
and Morris 1991

3.32 Low birthweight: area deprivation category, Scotland 1980–2

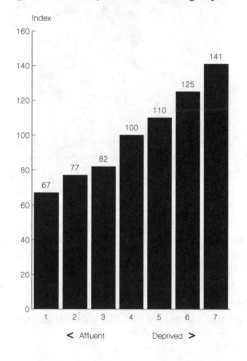

Source: Carstairs
and Morris 1991

Births under 2500 g

102

Geographical inequality and its socioeconomic causes can be examined in more detail by using smaller areas. A comparison of local government wards in Scotland showed that mortality increased with deprivation. Classification of areas was based on overcrowding, male unemployment, low social class and not having a car; category 1 is the most affluent and category 7 the most deprived. Infant mortality and the proportion of births weighing under 2500 g showed gradients with higher rates in the most deprived areas.

3.33 Mortality ratios: area deprivation category, Scotland 1980–2

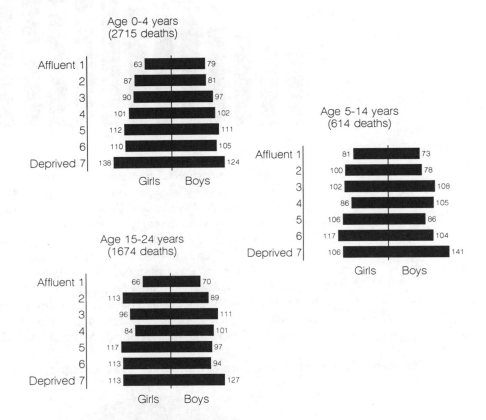

Source: Carstairs and Morris 1991

Mortality ratios for 0–4 year olds showed a clear gradient. Although ratios for 5–14 and 15–24 year olds were not as consistent (probably because of the smaller number of deaths), they still showed more favourable ratios in affluent areas. Mortality ratios express the rate for each deprivation category compared with the overall rate for the relevant age and sex; under 100 indicates lower than average mortality and over 100 higher than average (Carstairs and Morris 1991).

Homelessness

3.34 Trend in households accepted by local authorities as homeless, England 1978–90

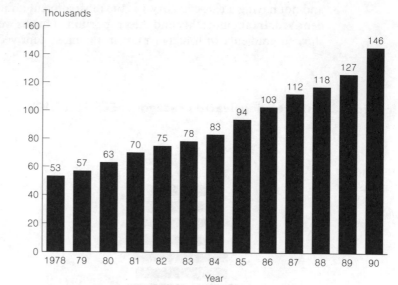

Thousands

Source: DoE 1979–91

Year

The only official measure of homelessness is the number of households accepted for rehousing by local authorities. In England 145,800 families were officially homeless in 1990, more than two-and-a-half times the 53,100 households homeless when the current system of counting began in 1978 (DoE 1979–91). Local authorities only accept as homeless about half the applications they receive. Trends in the rest of the UK have been similar.

A major factor in the dramatic rise in homelessness is the virtual disappearance of affordable rented housing. The private rented sector now provides less than 10 percent of housing, while council house building has been virtually frozen since 1979 (Greve and Currie 1990). Since 1990 the contribution of mortgage repossessions to homelessness has increased.

3.35 Households accepted as homeless: priority need category, Great Britain 1990

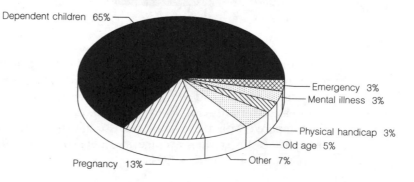

Dependent children 65%
Emergency 3%
Mental illness 3%
Physical handicap 3%
Old age 5%
Other 7%
Pregnancy 13%

Source: CSO Social Trends 21

104

In 1990 local authorities in Great Britain accepted 155,700 households as homeless and in priority need; that is, entitled to temporary accommodation and rehousing. Two-thirds of these were families with dependent children. An additional 13,800 households not in the priority need categories were also accepted as homeless (CSO Social Trends 21). The total number of households accepted as homeless represents more than 400,000 people, including around 200,000 dependent children.

Homeless single people are eligible for help only if they are 'vulnerable' because of, for example, mental illness. At least 156,000 young people under the age of 26 were estimated to be homeless in the UK in 1990 (Greve and Currie 1990). A survey in London estimated 51,000 homeless 16–19 year olds in London in 1987 (Ward 1990). The exact number is unknown, but efforts were made to include all homeless people in the 1991 Census.

3.36 Households in temporary accommodation with no play space, England and Wales 1987

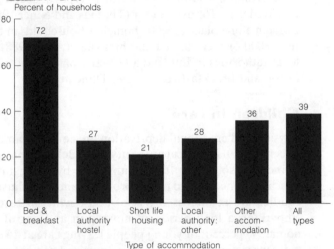

Source: Thomas and Niner 1989

Thirty-nine percent of all families with children in temporary accommodation in 1987 had no play space, indoor or outdoor, for their children – rising to 72 percent of households in bed and breakfast hostels (Thomas and Niner 1989). Overcrowding was a major problem: a fifth of children shared a bed with another child or an adult.

Inadequate and unsafe facilities for storage and preparation of food make some families depend on convenience foods and probably contribute to a high incidence of diarrhoea and vomiting. A high accident rate is also associated with inadequate cooking facilities. Long-term health consequences of home-lessness are difficult to monitor, but there is evidence that in addition to short-term gastrointestinal and respiratory infections, the stresses and poor environment may lead to behavioural problems and developmental delay (Wilson and Jenkins 1985; Drennan and Stearn 1986; Stearn 1986; HVA and BMA 1989).

3.37 Temporary accommodation occupied by households with children, England and Wales 1987

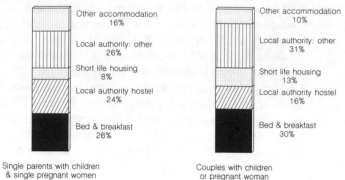

Other accommodation 16%

Local authority: other 26%

Short life housing 8%

Local authority hostel 24%

Bed & breakfast 26%

Single parents with children & single pregnant women

Other accommodation 10%

Local authority: other 31%

Short life housing 13%

Local authority hostel 16%

Bed & breakfast 30%

Couples with children or pregnant woman

Source: Thomas and Niner 1989

In 1987 the average length of stay of families in bed and breakfast was 21 weeks, compared with 33 weeks for all types of accommodation, but 7 percent had lived there for over a year (Thomas and Niner 1989). Local authorities in London alone placed 19,000 homeless households in temporary accommodation, 8000 of them in bed and breakfast (ALA 1988). Sixty-seven percent of local authorities in England and Wales place some of their homeless families in bed and breakfast (Evans and Duncan 1988).

Children in care

Physical and emotional deprivation are common among children at the time of being taken into local authority care (Bebbington and Miles 1989). The life chances of some are further impaired by being in care, leading to poor education, uncorrected health problems and maladjustment (DH 1991). Some children are at increased risk of abuse while in care (Dillner 1992). Many embark on a long period of moving in and out of institutions and foster homes: 40 percent of young people leaving care at 16 or over have had five or more placements in care. Homelessness and unemployment are common soon after leaving care (DH 1991). Thirty-seven percent of all young offenders are drawn either from those in care or from those who have recently left care.

There were 59,800 children and teenagers in local authority care in England in March 1991. The rate fell from 7.6 per 1000 children under 18 years old in 1981 to 5.5 in 1991. Children taken into care during the year (as opposed to children in care at year end) decreased in the same period from 3.1 to 2.7 per 1000 population under 18 (DH 1993). The fall results partly from policy changes, for example a shift away from taking the children of homeless families into care. The percentage of children in care who were in foster homes increased to 58 percent while community homes decreased to 16 percent.

The overall rate of children in care conceals a tenfold variation among local authorities, the highest rates being in the inner cities. Variation among local authorities likely to have similar levels of need points to differences in policy and resources.

3.38 Children in care: age, England March 1991

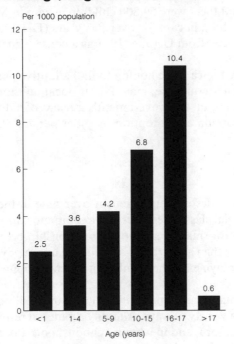

Per 1000 population

2.5 — <1
3.6 — 1-4
4.2 — 5-9
6.8 — 10-15
10.4 — 16-17
0.6 — >17

Age (years)

Source: DH 1993

3.39 Children in care: length of stay, England March 1991

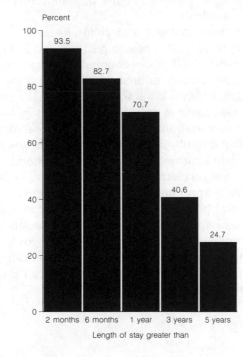

Percent

93.5 — 2 months
82.7 — 6 months
70.7 — 1 year
40.6 — 3 years
24.7 — 5 years

Length of stay greater than

Source: DH 1993

Total 59,800 children

107

Of all children in care 71 percent have spent more than a year of their lives this way. In England there were 59,800 children in care in March 1991, of whom 27 percent had been in care for over five years (DH 1992). The collection of these data changed from October 1991 as a consequence of the Children Act 1989.

Some children in care are hoping to find adoptive parents. The number of children in long-term care may fall if local authorities implement the recommendations of the government's review of adoption law, to allow inter-racial adoption and adoption by older parents (Dyer 1992).

Discussion

It is striking that despite improvement over time in the health of the whole population, social class differences still exist in mortality and morbidity at all ages. Statistics for small areas show a relationship between deprivation and mortality. More than a quarter of all children live in poverty, most because of parents' unemployment. The number of officially homeless families doubled in the last ten years.

Socioeconomic circumstances affect health in childhood, and probably also in later life, in a variety of ways. A family's material resources determine what housing it can afford, and in what neighbourhood. Poor housing conditions, poor local amenities and a generally more dangerous environment increase the risk of accidental death or injury to already disadvantaged sections of society (Chapter 4). Much of the higher child mortality in the manual social classes is due to accidents.

Proper nutrition of mothers and children depends on income to buy sufficient, healthy food, and access to healthy food in local shops. Cultural values are interwoven with socioeconomic circumstances, affecting family structures and lifestyles, such as breast-feeding and smoking habits (Chapter 5). Postneonatal mortality in lower social classes reflects not only poorer living conditions but also more maternal smoking than in higher social classes. Because of the interrelationships between different dimensions of social position it is often difficult to disentangle the pathways that affect health.

While exact causal pathways between socioeconomic circumstances and ill-health are not always clear, many of the health risks facing the disadvantaged are obvious and preventable. A common feature of these is that they are beyond the control both of the individuals affected and of health service professionals. Substantial improvement in the health of the children of disadvantaged communities requires action by government to improve employment opportunities and conditions, provide adequate social security benefits, and promote the availability of affordable, good quality housing and a safe environment for all children.

References

Publications other than routine data series

Association of London Authorities (1988) *Interim Working Party Report on Homelessness*. London, ALA.

Bebbington, A. and Miles, J. (1989) 'The background of children who enter local authority care', *British Journal of Social Work* 19(5): 349–68.

Butler, N. R. and Golding, J. (1986) *From Birth to Five*. Oxford, Pergamon Press.

Carstairs, V. and Morris, R. (1991) *Deprivation and Health in Scotland*. Aberdeen, Aberdeen University Press.

Davey Smith, G., Bartley, M. and Blane, D. (1990) 'The Black Report on socioeconomic inequalities in health 10 years on', *British Medical Journal* 301: 373–7.

Department of the Environment (1979–91) *Local Authority Action on Homelessness* (quarterly returns). London, HMSO.

Department of Health (1992) *Patterns and Outcomes in Child Placement: Messages from Current Research and Their Implications*. London, HMSO.

Department of Health (1993) *Personal Social Services: Local Authority Statistics. Children in Care of Local Authorities, Year Ending 31 March 1991, England (Provisional)*. London, DH.

Department of Health (Northern Ireland) (1991) *Personal Social Services Statistics for Northern Ireland, 1987*. Belfast, DH(NI).

Department of Health and Social Security (1976) *Sharing Resources for Health in England, Report of the Resource Allocation Working Party*. London, HMSO.

Department of Health and Social Security (1980) *Inequalities in Health: Report of a Research Working Group (the Black Report)*. London, DHSS.

Department of Social Security (1990) *Households below Average Income – a Statistical Analysis 1981–87*. London, HMSO.

Department of Social Security (1991) *Social Security Statistics 1990*. London, HMSO.

Dillner, L. (1992) 'Children at risk in homes', *British Medical Journal* 304: 403.

Drennan, V. and Stearn, J. (1986) 'Health visitors and homeless families', *Health Visitor* 59: 340–2.

Dyer, C. (1992) 'Children to get more say in adoptions', *Guardian* 20 October.

Evans, A. and Duncan S. (1988) *Responding to Homelessness: Local Authority Policy and Practice*. London, HMSO.

Greve, J. and Currie, E. (1990) *Homelessness in Britain*. York, Joseph Rowntree Memorial Trust.

Health Visitors Association and British Medical Association (1989) *Homeless Families and Their Health*. London, BMA.

House of Commons Social Services Committee (1990) *Households Below Average Income – a Regional Analysis 1980–85*. London, HMSO.

National Children's Home (1992) *The NCH Fact File – Children in Britain 1992*. London, NCH.

Oppenheim, C. (1990) *Poverty: the Facts*. London, Child Poverty Action Group.

Roll, J. (1990) *Young People: Growing up in the Welfare State*. London, Family Policy Studies Centre.

Scottish Education Department (1990) *Children in Care or Under Supervision*. Edinburgh, SED.

Smyth, M. and Robus, N. (1989) *The Financial Circumstances of Families with Disabled Children Living in Private Households*. OPCS Surveys of Disability in Great Britain, report 5. London, HMSO.

Stearn, J. (1986) 'An expensive way of making children ill', *Roof* October: 11–14.

Thomas, A. and Niner, P. (1989) *Living in Temporary Accommodation: a Survey of Homeless People*. London, HMSO.

Walker, A. (1982) *Unqualified and Underemployed: Handicapped Young People and the Labour Market*. London, Macmillan.

Ward, A. (1990) *Young and Homeless*. Fact sheet 2. London, Shelter.

Welsh Office (1991) *Child Protection Registers: Statistics for Wales 1990*. Cardiff, Welsh Office.

Whitehead, M. (1988) *The Health Divide*. Harmondsworth, Penguin.

Wilson, T. and Jenkins, S. (1985) 'The health of homeless families', Meeting of the Community Paediatric Research Group, London.

Routine data series

Office of Population Censuses and Surveys:
 OPCS DH3 Mortality statistics: perinatal and infant
 OPCS DS Occupational mortality
 OPCS FM1 Birth statistics
 OPCS GHS General Household Survey
 OPCS MB5 Morbidity statistics from general practice
 OPCS Monitors are periodic bulletins between the main volumes.
Central Statistical Office:
 CSO Social Trends

CHAPTER 4   Physical environment

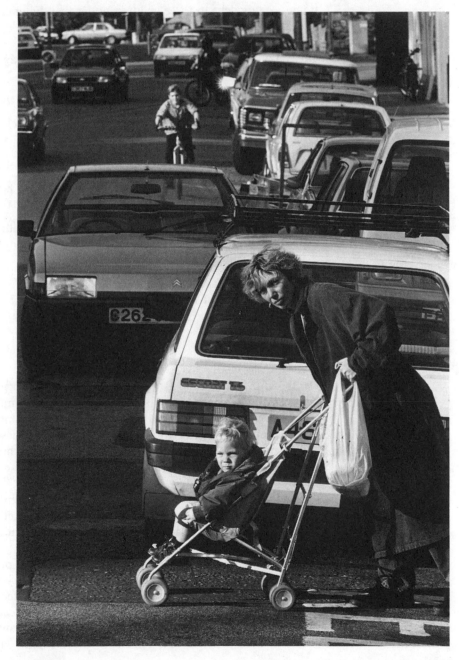

Key facts

- Accidents cause nearly one-half of all deaths for ages 1–19. They are also an important cause of morbidity and long-term disability.

- Over half of the fatal accidents to infants and children under five happen at home – equivalent to three children under five dying each week in the UK.

- Fires cause one-half of all home accident deaths.

- On average in the UK one child under 15 and two teenagers aged 15–19 die on the roads every day.

- The child pedestrian death rate in the UK is one of the highest in Europe.

- At all ages and for most types of accident boys have a higher death rate than girls.

- Some 4 percent of children live in housing officially considered unfit for use.

- Environmental tobacco smoke is the most important pollutant in the home. Passive smoking damages the health of children and the unborn fetus.

- Road traffic is an important source of outdoor air pollution. The density of traffic (measured in vehicle kilometres) is forecast to double by the year 2005.

- Pollution on a global scale, the thinning of the stratospheric ozone layer and global warming (through the greenhouse effect), threatens the health of children now and of future generations.

Introduction

Death during childhood is now rare, largely due to improvements in the physical environment – in housing, sanitation and nutrition – leading to control of the infectious diseases that were once major killers, such as cholera, typhoid and tuberculosis (McKeown 1979). Despite these improvements, the environment still presents threats to health. Further, in industrialized societies, the environmental hazards that children face are changing constantly.

Children are vulnerable to accidents in an environment built principally for adults. The average house is equipped with potentially lethal gadgets. Outside, traffic poses an obvious threat, with large numbers of children killed or injured in road accidents each week.

Traffic threatens health more insidiously through air pollution. Pollution of the air, soil, food and water also results from industry and farming, power stations and disposal of waste, which may be toxic, infectious or radioactive. The developing fetus, infants and children are physically more susceptible than adults to the harmful effects of many pollutants (BMA 1991). In addition, their lifestyle and behaviour may lead to greater exposure, for

112

example through playing in contaminated areas or eating soil. Breast-fed babies may be exposed to hazardous substances in their mother's milk.

Environmental hazards do not affect all children equally. Children are vulnerable to different hazards at different ages. Inquisitive toddlers are most at risk of accidents in the home. Road traffic accidents pose the greatest threat to older children. Primary school children are at particular risk as pedestrians, secondary school children on bicycles, and young adults on motorbikes or in cars. At all ages, and for most types of accidents, boys are more likely to have accidents than girls. Finally, a family's socioeconomic status will largely determine its material environment: the children of the poor are the most likely to live in inadequate housing and, with nowhere else to play, end up unsupervised in the street. They are more likely to live in areas with high levels of air pollution, close to industrial estates or busy traffic. They are also more likely to be subjected to what is probably the most harmful common pollutant, environmental tobacco smoke.

Accidents

The importance of injuries as a cause of death and morbidity has been described in Chapter 2. The majority of injuries are unintentional – the result of accidents. Accidents cause 43 percent of deaths for ages 1–19 (England and Wales 1987–90). The term 'accident' suggests that these injuries are largely inevitable and the result of 'bad luck'. But accidents are not random events. They occur in predictable patterns. These patterns and their implications for prevention are outlined in this chapter.

For every child who dies, many more suffer non-fatal injuries. The Child Accident Prevention Trust estimates that in England and Wales around 120,000 children under 15 are admitted to hospital following an accident each year, and about two million attend an accident and emergency department (CAPT 1989). Many injured children are dealt with by their general practitioner without ever attending hospital. Over the three-year period 1987–9, 5 percent of children under 16 had had an accident requiring medical attention in the three months prior to interview. Of these, 19 percent of 0–4 year olds and 15 percent of 5–15 year olds consulted their family doctor only (OPCS GHS 17–19).

Injuries can leave residual disability in any area of functioning, from physical (e.g. deformity), neurological (e.g. epilepsy, paralysis) and sensory (e.g. blindness), to psychological, behavioural and social. The extent to which injuries cause disability is not known, but a few studies provide estimates. One widely quoted small-scale study estimated that around 3 percent of children under 15 years admitted to hospital after an accident are left with a permanent disability (Avery and Gibbs 1985), while national data from a large birth cohort show that, for 16–23 year olds, a permanent disability results from at least 9 percent of accidents resulting in admission to hospital and 2 percent of those prompting attendance at a casualty department (M. Barker and C. Power, unpublished data).

4.1 Change in mortality from accidents: age and sex, England 1969 and 1990

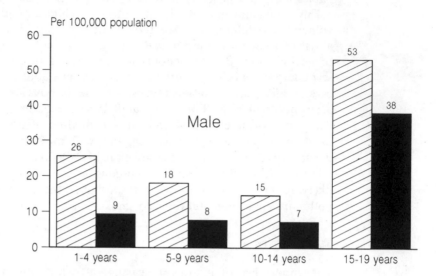

Per 100,000 population

Male

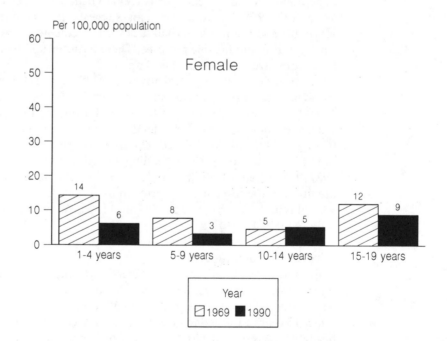

Per 100,000 population

Female

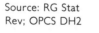

Year
▨ 1969 ■ 1990

Source: RG Stat
Rev; OPCS DH2

ICD codes E800–949

Accident death rates improved between 1969 and 1990 for all age groups except 10–14 year old girls. Mortality for males is consistently higher than for females.

4.2 Type of fatal accident: age, England and Wales 1987–90

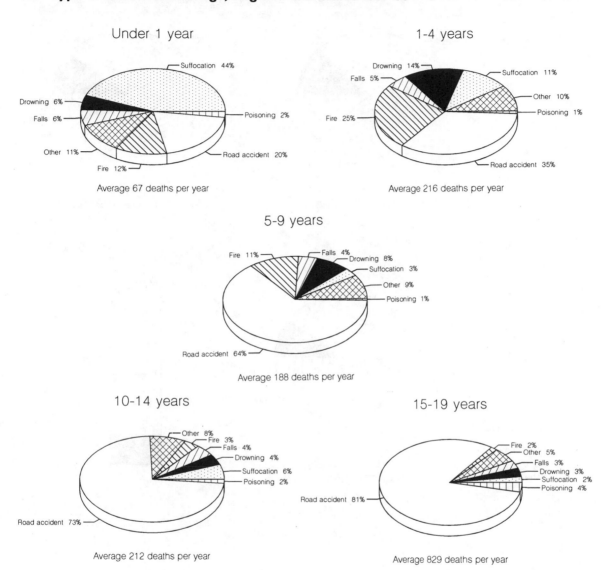

Under 1 year

- Suffocation 44%
- Poisoning 2%
- Road accident 20%
- Fire 12%
- Other 11%
- Falls 6%
- Drowning 6%

Average 67 deaths per year

1-4 years

- Drowning 14%
- Falls 5%
- Fire 25%
- Suffocation 11%
- Other 10%
- Poisoning 1%
- Road accident 35%

Average 216 deaths per year

5-9 years

- Fire 11%
- Falls 4%
- Drowning 8%
- Suffocation 3%
- Other 9%
- Poisoning 1%
- Road accident 64%

Average 188 deaths per year

10-14 years

- Other 8%
- Fire 3%
- Falls 4%
- Drowning 4%
- Suffocation 6%
- Poisoning 2%
- Road accident 73%

Average 212 deaths per year

15-19 years

- Fire 2%
- Other 5%
- Falls 3%
- Drowning 3%
- Suffocation 2%
- Poisoning 4%
- Road accident 81%

Average 829 deaths per year

Source: OPCS DH2

The causes of accidental injury at different ages reflect both stage of development and exposure to different environmental hazards during different periods of childhood. This is most strikingly demonstrated by the increasing dominance of road accidents as a cause of fatal injury as children get older. Conversely, children spend less time at home as they grow up, so that deaths caused by fires, an important cause of death in the home, become less common.

115

4.3 Deaths from accidents at home: age and cause, England and Wales 1987–90

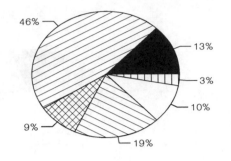

46%
13%
3%
10%
19%
9%

Infants under 1 year
Annual mean 39 deaths

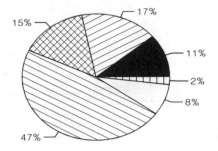

15%
17%
11%
2%
8%
47%

1-4 years
Annual mean 109 deaths

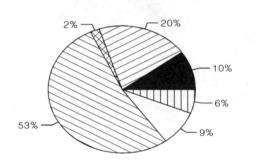

2%
20%
10%
6%
9%
53%

5-14 years
Annual mean 48 deaths

Source: OPCS DH4

ICD E850–949
excluding those
outside the home

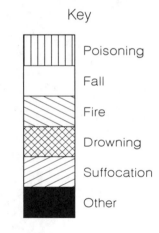

Key

Poisoning

Fall

Fire

Drowning

Suffocation

Other

Over half the fatal accidents in infants and pre-school children happen at home, equivalent to three children under five dying each week. Once school age is reached, the proportion of accidental deaths that take place in the home falls to one in eight as deaths due to road accidents increase.

Fire is the most common cause of accidental death at home, and accounts for one-half of these deaths among children aged 1–14. In 1990, fire caused 98 deaths among those under the age of 20, and two-thirds (49) of these were children under five. Younger children are at particular risk in house fires because they are not able to make their own escape.

4.4 Non-fatal injuries from fire: age and sex, United Kingdom 1990

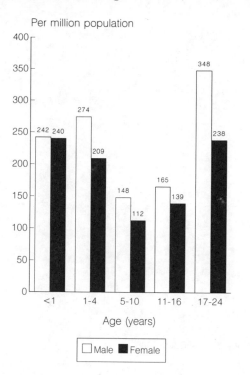

Per million population

Age (years)

☐ Male ■ Female

Source: Home Office
1992

The Home Office publishes statistics about fires attended by fire brigades in the United Kingdom. These complement the statistics of OPCS and the Scottish and Northern Irish Registrar Generals but cannot be directly compared. The Home Office statistics give some indication of the considerable number of children who suffer non-fatal injuries in fires. The majority of these are house fires: of 4206 casualties among under 24 year olds in 1990, 93 percent were in buildings, mostly homes. At each age there are more male casualties than female, particularly among 17–24 year olds. This age group also has the highest non-fatal fire casualty rate of any age.

It should be noted that Home Office figures do not include children injured in fires put out without the fire brigade being called.

The Home Office statistics also give details of the source of ignition and nature of injury. The number of fires started by smokers is increasing. Of the 64,200 house fires attended by the fire brigade in 1990, 12 percent were started by smokers' materials. However, they accounted for 40 percent of the 627 house fires in which a death (any age) occurred.

Over half (56 percent) of the deaths (any age) in house fires are solely from inhaling smoke, and one-fifth from burns alone. One-third of non-fatal casualties are overcome by smoke or gas and one-fifth are burnt. Smoke detectors are associated with faster fire discovery times and a lower death rate.

117

4.5 Trend in accidental house fires caused by smokers' materials, United Kingdom 1981–90

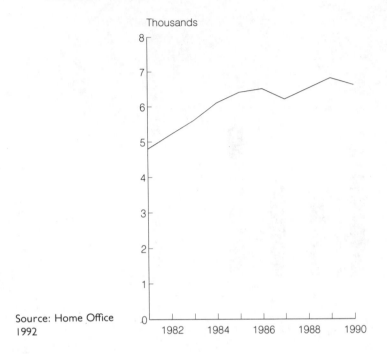

Thousands

Source: Home Office 1992

4.6 Non-fatal accidents* at home: age and cause, United Kingdom 1989

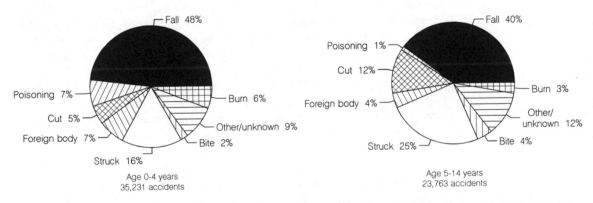

Fall 48%

Poisoning 7%

Cut 5%

Foreign body 7%

Struck 16%

Bite 2%

Other/unknown 9%

Burn 6%

Age 0-4 years
35,231 accidents

Fall 40%

Poisoning 1%

Cut 12%

Foreign body 4%

Struck 25%

Bite 4%

Other/unknown 12%

Burn 3%

Age 5-14 years
23,763 accidents

Source: DTI 1992

*Presenting at hospital accident departments

The Department of Trade and Industry, through its Home Accident Surveillance System (HASS), collects information about non-fatal injuries resulting from home accidents, based on attendances at the accident departments of a sample of 22 hospitals in the UK.

Although fires are the major cause of accidental death at home, burns account for only 5 percent of non-fatal home accidents, and only 3 percent of

118

non-fatal burns are the result of a house fire. The type of burn varies with age (CAPT 1985). Toddlers and young children are most likely to be scalded by spilled hot drinks, or hot water from a kettle or overturned saucepan. In 1989, it was estimated from the HASS sample that over 32,000 children under five were brought to an accident department after a scald at home. They also typically get contact burns from hot surfaces, such as irons and cookers (there were just over 21,000 attendances for other burns). Older children are burned playing with matches and lighters, while adolescents, especially boys, experiment with outdoor fires, often using flammable liquids.

Childhood accidental poisoning is mainly a problem of one and two year olds, who are inquisitive and oral, and have an apparent lack of concern for unpleasant taste. Most poisonings take place in the home. They are rarely fatal (a total of eight deaths in children under 15 in England and Wales in 1990). Although poisoning accounts for a small proportion of casualty attendances following a home accident, a relatively large number of pre-school children are admitted to hospital with poisoning. In 1985 in England an estimated 12,000 children under five were admitted following poisoning – a quarter of all hospital admissions following an accident.

Medicines are involved in three-quarters of fatal poisonings in children (Craft 1983) and one half of casualty attendances (Burger 1984). Household products cause most of the remaining cases. The packaging, prescribing and storage of medicines are clearly important ways of influencing the risk of childhood poisoning.

A larger number of teenagers aged 15–19 die through poisoning (37 in 1990). It is likely that a proportion of these deaths were actually suicides. Since the mid-1980s there has been an increase in poisoning deaths due to inhalation of solvents and bottled gas (see Chapter 5).

4.7   Falls in the home: type, age 0–14, United Kingdom 1989

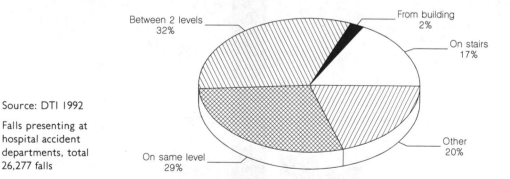

Source: DTI 1992

Falls presenting at hospital accident departments, total 26,277 falls

Falls are the most common type of home accident, although they account for a relatively small proportion of deaths. Two-thirds of falls in the 0–14 group occur in the under fives. There is scope for prevention through safe housing design, use of stair gates and window locks.

119

4.8   Trend in road traffic accident deaths: age, Great Britain 1970–91

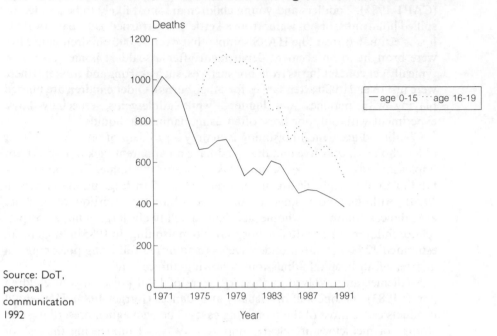

Source: DoT,
personal
communication
1992

**4.9   Deaths from road traffic accidents: age, England and Wales, annual average
1987–90**

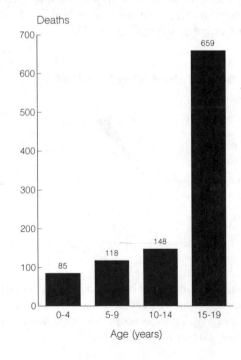

Source: OPCS DH2

ICD codes E800–949

120

An increase in motor vehicles has coincided with a decrease in road traffic accident deaths. From 1970 to 1990 deaths of 0–15 year olds from road traffic accidents fell by 59 percent while the flow of motor vehicles increased by 72 percent (CSO Social Trends 22).

In 1990 in the United Kingdom, 387 children under 15 and 725 young adults aged 15–19 were killed in road traffic accidents. This means on average one child under 15 and two 15–19 year olds dying each day (OPCS DH2/17). The rates are 3 per 100,000 in pre-school children, 4 in children of 5–14 years and 19 for the 15–19 age group.

4.10 Children aged 0–14 injured in road traffic accidents: severity of injury and type of road user, Great Britain 1990

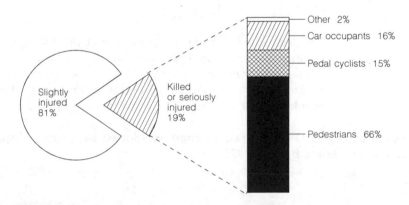

Other 2%

Car occupants 16%

Pedal cyclists 15%

Pedestrians 66%

Slightly injured 81%

Killed or seriously injured 19%

Source: DoT
Casualty Report 1992

Total 48,853 children

The Department of Transport publishes statistics on road accidents in Great Britain occurring on the public highway and reported to the police. These statistics complement those published by OPCS and the Scottish Registrar General but are not directly comparable.

In 1990, 368 children were killed in road accidents, 299 as pedestrians. Pedestrians make up two-thirds of all fatal and serious injuries to children on the road. Two-thirds of these pedestrian casualties are boys. Over five times as many boys as girls are killed or seriously injured in bicycle accidents (DoT 1992). In contrast, equal numbers are injured as passengers in a car.

For school children, a quarter of all injuries happen on the way to or, more commonly, from school. The majority of road accidents involving children on foot or on a bike happen on residential roads carrying only light traffic (DoT 1992).

4.11 Child pedestrian mortality age 0–14, Europe 1989

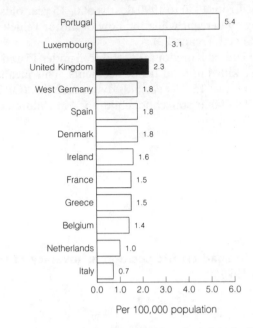

Source: DoT,
personal
communication
1992

Per 100,000 population

The death rate for child pedestrians in the United Kingdom, at 2.3 per 100,000 children under 15 in 1989, was one of the worst in Europe (European Community average in 1989 was 1.7). This is despite the fact that the death rate for all child road users was one of the lowest. In 1989 the UK child road accident death rate was 3.7, compared with the EC average of 4.4

4.12 Teenagers aged 15–19 injured in road accidents: severity of injury and type of road user, Great Britain 1990

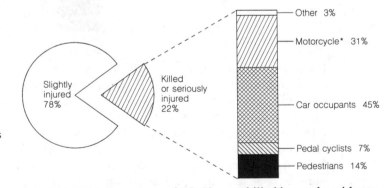

Source: DoT
Casualty Report 1992

Total 57,885 teenagers
*Includes all
two-wheeled
motorized vehicles

In 1990, 678 teenagers aged 15–19 were killed in road accidents, an average of one every day in a car and one every two days on a motorbike. Nearly three-quarters of the 33,166 car drivers under 20 involved in a road accident with a casualty were men. Of the motorbike, scooter or moped riders under 20 years of age, 90 percent were men.

4.13 Rate of road traffic deaths and serious injuries: age and type of road user, Great Britain 1990

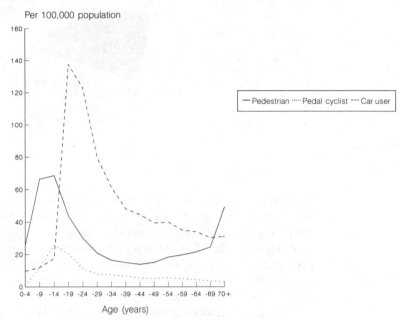

Per 100,000 population

Legend: — Pedestrian ····· Pedal cyclist --- Car user

Age (years)

Source: DoT
Casualty Report 1992

4.14 Rate of deaths and serious injuries in motorbike riders: age, Great Britain 1990

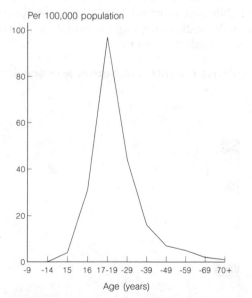

Per 100,000 population

Age (years)

Source: DoT
Casualty Report 1992

Because not all road accidents that cause injury are reported to the police, these figures are known to underestimate the true number of casualties. This is especially true for cycle accidents.

123

4.15   Deaths from accidents other than road traffic: cause, age 1–19, England and Wales 1987–90

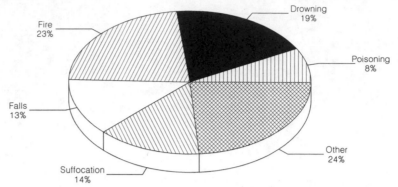

Fire
23%

Drowning
19%

Poisoning
8%

Falls
13%

Other
24%

Suffocation
14%

Source: OPCS DH2

Annual mean 420 deaths

Drowning accounts for a fifth of all accidental death other than road traffic accidents in children and young adults. In the two year period 1988–9 there were 149 drownings and 157 near drownings (i.e. asphyxia after submersion) of children under 15 in the UK. The estimated annual rate of submersion accidents is 1.5 per 100,000, with mortality of 0.7 per 100,000. The overall boy to girl ratio is 3 : 1, and boys under five have the highest rate (3.6 per 100,000) (Kemp and Sibert 1992).

The type of accident depends largely on age. Babies and toddlers drown in the bath, mostly when left unsupervised. Toddlers and small children fall in garden ponds and domestic swimming pools. School children drown in open waterways (rivers, canals, lakes), the sea and swimming pools. Of the 33 accidents in public swimming pools only two (6 percent) were fatal; however, half of those in domestic swimming pools and over three-quarters of those in open waterways resulted in death.

4.16   Non-fatal non-traffic accidents outside the home: age and location, United Kingdom 1989

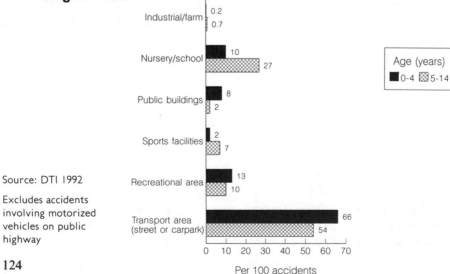

Source: DTI 1992

Excludes accidents involving motorized vehicles on public highway

Per 100 accidents

124

The Leisure Accident Surveillance System (LASS), run by the Department of Trade and Industry, collects information on accidents occurring outside the home, not including those that involve motor vehicles on the public highway, but covering, for example, bicycle accidents in which a motor vehicle was not involved. Most of these accidents take place in a 'transport area' (street or car park).

For 5–14 year olds, school is the next most common place. Just over half the accidents at school (58 percent in 1987) are to boys. Accidents most commonly happen at play (37 percent in 1987), the commonest type being a fall (33 percent). Only 2 percent of cases require admission to hospital.

Schools are required to send details of accidents to local education authorities, but these data are not made available for analysis or collated centrally.

For the under fives, the second most common place for a non-traffic accident outside the home is a recreational area – mostly playgrounds and parks or the countryside. Three-quarters of playground accidents involve children aged 5–14. Over two-thirds of these accidents are to boys. The most common type of accident is a fall, most often between two levels. Swings and climbing frames are the equipment most often involved. Of children injured in playgrounds, 5 percent are admitted to hospital as inpatients (DTI 1990).

The home environment

4.17 Damp housing and illness among 10 year olds, United Kingdom 1980

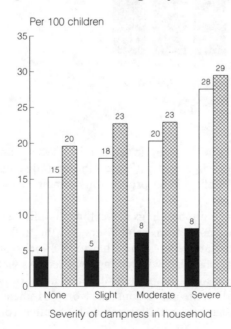

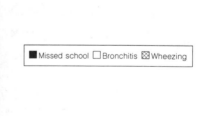

Source: Child Health and Education Survey, unpublished

125

Children living in damp homes have more respiratory symptoms, headaches and fever, and are more likely to miss school, than those living in drier conditions. Of 10 year olds living in homes with severe dampness, 8 percent missed school, compared with only 4 percent of those in homes with no damp. Dampness, particularly condensation, harbours fungi and other organisms. Temperature and humidity affect the level of fungal spores and house dust mite antigen in the air. It is possible that such factors contribute to the onset of childhood respiratory diseases, such as asthma (Lowry 1991).

4.18 Households living in damp or unfit dwellings: age of youngest child, England 1986

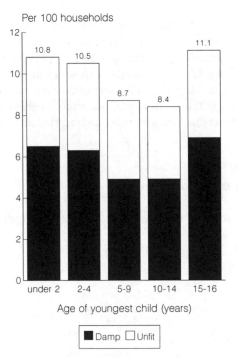

Source: DoE Housing
Condition Survey,
unpublished

A national survey of housing in England in 1986 found that 6 percent of households with a child under 17 lived in damp dwellings and 4 percent in housing deemed unfit. These proportions remained relatively constant for children of all ages.

Many cheaply built buildings have flimsy walls and inadequate sound insulation, so that noise from neighbours and the traffic outside can disturb sleep and lead to family stress and tensions. Blocks of flats are often not suitable homes for families with young children. As well as the question of safety, they can be socially isolating. In many areas of poor housing, fear of crime and vandalism are also a constant worry. Homeless families housed in bed and breakfast accommodation are likely to suffer from all these problems.

The effects of poor housing are likely to be compounded by the other consequences of poverty described in Chapter 3.

4.19 Sources of indoor air pollution

Source	Pollutant
Cigarettes, cigars etc.	Environmental tobacco smoke
Heating and cooking appliances	Carbon monoxide, nitrogen dioxide
Biological agents	Infection, allergens, irritant biological material
Building products	Formaldehyde, volatile organic compounds, lead, fibres
Subsoil	Radon, methane
DIY, hobbies	Volatile organic compounds

Source: BMA 1990

The air inside a house may be more polluted than that outdoors. This is important because children spend much of their time indoors. In the 1950s an average room had around ten air changes an hour. Now, with better insulation, there may be less than one. Even pollutants that have a weak effect may be important because of the large numbers of children exposed.

High levels of nitrogen dioxide can form during cooking on a gas stove. Peak concentrations in a kitchen can reach those at the kerbside of a busy road (DoE, personal communication). Nitrogen dioxide is a respiratory irritant and increases the risk of respiratory infection. In children with asthma, it may increase the frequency and severity of asthma attacks. There is evidence of a higher prevalence of childhood respiratory symptoms in homes with a gas cooker, possibly due to nitrogen dioxide (Read 1991).

Carbon monoxide is also a product of gas cookers and heaters. During cooking levels are often above those in urban areas with heavy traffic. However, when a gas oven is used for heating, which is common in poorer households, levels may be five times higher than in a busy street (DoE, personal communication). Carbon monoxide reduces the oxygen carrying capacity of the blood, causing neurological symptoms such as headaches and drowsiness. There is also evidence of cardiovascular effects, even at relatively low levels. Exposure to carbon monoxide during pregnancy can retard fetal growth (Read 1991).

A report by the Royal College of Physicians summarizes what is known about the harmful effects of passive smoking on the health of children, including the unborn fetus (RCP 1992):

Passive smoking and the health of the fetus

- Babies born to mothers who smoke are lighter by an average 200 grams (approximately half a pound). Paternal smoking also makes babies significantly lighter.
- Spontaneous abortions (miscarriages) of viable fetuses are increased in pregnant smokers by more than one-quarter (approximately equivalent to 4300 miscarriages per year in England and Wales).
- Premature labour is twice as common in pregnant smokers.
- Perinatal mortality (stillbirths and early neonatal deaths) is increased by approximately one-third in babies of smokers. This is equivalent to approximately 420 deaths per year in England and Wales.
- The effects of smoking in pregnancy extend well beyond infancy, with a reduction in growth and educational achievement.

Passive smoking and the health of children

- Children of parents who smoke inhale nicotine in amounts equivalent to their actively smoking 60–150 cigarettes per year.
- Over one-quarter of the risk of death due to sudden infant death syndrome (cot death) is attributable to maternal smoking (equivalent to 365 deaths per year in England and Wales).
- Infants of parents who smoke are twice as likely to suffer from serious respiratory infection.
- Symptoms of asthma are twice as common in the children of smokers.
- One-third of cases of 'glue ear', the commonest cause of deafness in children, are attributable to parental smoking.
- Children of parents who smoke more than 10 cigarettes per day tend to be shorter than children of non-smokers.
- Passive smoking is an important cause of school absenteeism, accounting for one in seven days lost.
- Parental smoking is responsible for at least 17,000 admissions to hospital each year of children under the age of five.
- Passive smoking during childhood predisposes children to develop chronic obstructive airways disease and cancer as adults.
- Maternal smoking during pregnancy and infancy is one of the most important avoidable risk factors for infant death.

The increased exposure to nicotine among children whose parents smoke may be measured indirectly by the amount of cotinine in a child's saliva. Cotinine is produced from nicotine, and cotinine levels in children have been found to be closely related to levels of nicotine measured in the air at home. In children who are not themselves smokers, cotinine levels are over four times as high when both parents smoke as when neither parent does so. From the data on cotinine levels, it has been estimated that children of parents who smoke receive a total dose of nicotine equivalent to their actively smoking 60 to 150 cigarettes a year (RCP 1992).

4.20 Cotinine in non-smoking 11–15 year olds: parental smoking, England 1990

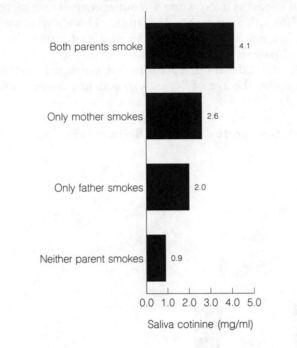

Both parents smoke — 4.1

Only mother smokes — 2.6

Only father smokes — 2.0

Neither parent smokes — 0.9

0.0 1.0 2.0 3.0 4.0 5.0

Saliva cotinine (mg/ml)

Source: Lader and
Matheson 1991

4.21 Smoking by married parents living with children: parental age and sex, Great Britain 1990

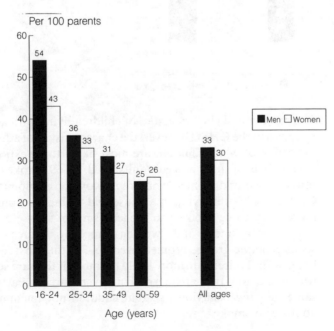

Per 100 parents

■ Men □ Women

16-24: 54, 43
25-34: 36, 33
35-49: 31, 27
50-59: 25, 26
All ages: 33, 30

Age (years)

Source: OPCS GHS 21

129

A third of married men living with dependent children are smokers (1988 data) and almost as many women. Younger parents are more likely to smoke, over half the fathers under age 25 doing so. This is important because younger children are more vulnerable to the effects of passive smoking. Data for unmarried parents are not available.

The Health Education Authority has estimated that four million UK children under the age of 10 are exposed to passive smoking (Mihill and Linton 1992).

4.22 Smoking: economic status age 16–59, Great Britain 1990

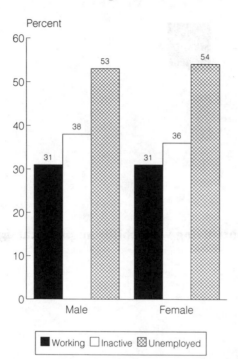

Source: OPCS GHS 21

The number and characteristics of children living with adults who smoke are not given in the GHS. However, the characteristics of adult smokers give some indication of which children are most likely to be exposed.

Over half of unemployed adults aged 16–59 smoke, compared to only a third of men and women who are in work or economically inactive (OPCS GHS 21). Children living in a household with an unemployed adult are thus more likely to be exposed to tobacco smoke.

For both men and women smoking increases with decreasing socioeconomic group. Women aged 25–34 (the most likely age group to be living with children) are more likely to smoke if they are separated, divorced or widowed than if they are married or never married. Partners tend to have the same smoking behaviour, so that children not uncommonly live with two adults who smoke.

4.23 Sources of exposure to radiation, United Kingdom 1991

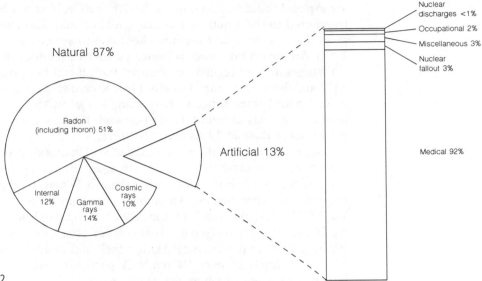

Source: DoE 1992

In the United Kingdom, the annual average dose from background radiation is about 2.5 mSv per person. Most comes from natural sources: the sun and outer space (cosmic), soil and building materials (gamma radiation and radon), and the natural radioactivity of the body. Radon, from uranium, and its principal isotope thoron are the most damaging to health: they are inhaled and are a potential cause of lung cancer (Lowry 1991). Outdoors, radon gas is diluted and concentrations are low. But with current standards of insulation, radon that seeps into houses can build up to high levels.

Around 100,000 homes in England (0.5 percent of the total) are estimated to have concentrations that are above the government's 'action level' of $200 \, Bq/m^3$ (NRPB 1992). Most are in Devon and Cornwall. The average dose of radon to people living in Cornwall is three times the UK average. Although it has been estimated that radon in homes may cause about 2000 cases of lung cancer a year (one in 20 cases), this is based on the effects of very high doses on uranium miners. There is little direct evidence that the lower levels found in houses cause lung cancer (Lowry 1991).

Lead is poisonous, particularly to the central nervous system. Young children are vulnerable because their brain is still developing, and chronic exposure to low levels of lead can impair mental development (CEH/CAPP 1987; FoE 1990b; Read 1991; Godlee and Walker 1992). The DoE has a higher threshold

131

for blood lead concentration than do the regulations in France and the USA. The upper limit is 25 mg per 100 ml in Britain and 10 mg in France. Children are exposed to lead in food and water, as well as in soil, which tends to be transferred to the mouth at this age. Children may also chew old toys and paint that contain lead (new household paint has been lead-free only since 1987). An important source is leaded petrol (see outdoor pollution).

Changes in food regulations reduced the general limit of lead in food in 1979, and the level in canned food in 1985. Recent analyses of the lead content in food in the United Kingdom have found low levels: the average intake from food in 1989 was around 0.11 mg per week for children, a fall of about 5 percent since the mid-1970s (MAFF 1989).

Lead water pipes are the main source of lead in drinking water. In 1982 the Government estimated that 8.5 million households in England and Wales still had lead plumbing (FoE 1990a). An estimated 34 percent of primary schools were built at a time when lead plumbing would have been used (FoE 1990b). The 1992 WHO guidelines for the maximum amount of lead in drinking water are 10 parts per billion (p.p.b.). However, of samples taken in England and Wales in 1990, 19 percent exceeded this limit and some children are drinking water with levels of over 100 p.p.b. A particular risk-group is bottle-fed infants, 90 percent of whose diet is tap water.

The outdoor environment

The 1956 Clean Air Act led to a marked improvement in the level of air pollution from the burning of coal (sulphur dioxide and black smoke) and has put an end to the winter smogs that were once an annual occurrence. However, air quality is again worsening, mainly as a result of the increasing volume of road traffic, and summer 'photochemical' smogs have become a feature of cities around the country (Read 1991; Godlee and Walker 1992). This new pollution is a 'cocktail' of chemicals, whose exact effects on health are not known.

The major effects of air pollutants are respiratory, and children who already have a respiratory illness are particularly vulnerable (Read 1991). This is important because asthma is the commonest chronic illness in childhood (Chapter 2). The question as to whether rising levels of air pollution are responsible for the recently observed increase in the prevalence and severity of asthma attacks in childhood remains to be answered (Anonymous 1990).

Exposure to air pollution as a child may cause illness in adulthood. Recurrent respiratory illness and impaired lung function in childhood are important factors in the development of adult chronic obstructive airways disease (Strachan 1992). Cancer caused by exposure to potential carcinogens, such as benzene, may take many years to develop (Godlee and Walker 1992).

The adverse health effects of sulphurous pollution have long been recognized. In children, acute exposure is associated with irritation of the eyes and respiratory system, and with an increased risk of respiratory infections. It causes wheezing in children with asthma. Long-term exposure increases the prevalence of and mortality from asthma and bronchitis (Read 1991; Godlee and Walker 1992).

Sulphur dioxide emissions fell by 23 percent between 1980 and 1990. Power stations are the main source (72 percent in 1990). Although there has been an overall decrease in black smoke emissions of 19 percent over the decade, the contribution from diesel-powered vehicles, the main source, rose by 75 percent (DoE 1992).

The 1983 EC Directives for sulphur dioxide, generally regarded as lax, are regularly breached in Belfast. The more stringent WHO guidelines are exceeded more widely throughout the United Kingdom. Adverse health effects to children have been demonstrated at levels within these guidelines.

Globally, sulphur dioxide levels are rising, and in Eastern Europe and the Third World sulphurous pollution remains a serious threat to health. Sulphur dioxide is the main constituent of acid rain, which causes environmental damage by acidifying lakes and other surface water and by killing trees and vegetation.

4.24   Trend in nitrogen oxide emissions: source, United Kingdom 1980–90

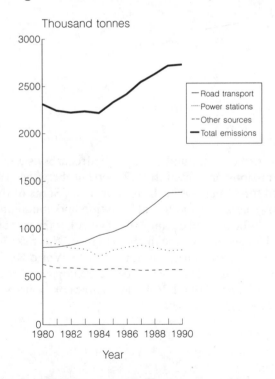

Source: DoE 1992

In 1990, 51 percent of nitrogen oxide pollution came from road traffic. Whereas emissions from other sources declined between 1980 and 1990, those from road transport rose by 72 percent. Of the nitrogen oxides, nitrogen

133

dioxide is the most harmful to human health (see section on indoor air quality). Nitrogen oxides contribute to the formation of ozone, a harmful secondary pollutant. Nitrogen dioxide is a cause of acid rain.

4.25 Trend in volatile organic compound emissions: source, United Kingdom 1980–90

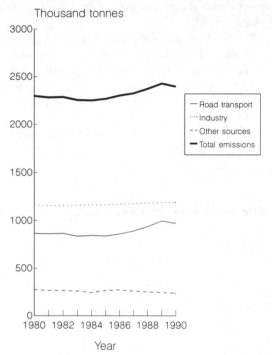

Thousand tonnes

Road transport
Industry
Other sources
Total emissions

Year

Source: DoE 1992

Volatile organic compounds, such as hydrocarbons and benzene, from road traffic emissions increased by 12 percent between 1980 and 1990, and accounted for 41 percent of the total in 1990. Some of these compounds can cause drowsiness, eye and throat irritation and coughing. In terms of known health effects benzene, a component of petrol, is the most harmful. It is known to cause leukaemia. Although the extent of the risk of cancer to children through exposure to benzene is not clear, the World Health Organisation has stated that because it is known to be a carcinogen, there can be no 'safe' level (Godlee and Walker 1992). Volatile organic compounds are directly involved in the formation of ozone.

Sunlight acting on a mixture of nitrogen oxides, oxygen and volatile organic compounds forms ozone, a major component of summer smogs. At low concentrations ozone is an irritant to the eyes, nose and throat, and causes

4.26 Number of hours in which average ozone exceeded 80 p.p.b., British Isles annual average 1987–90

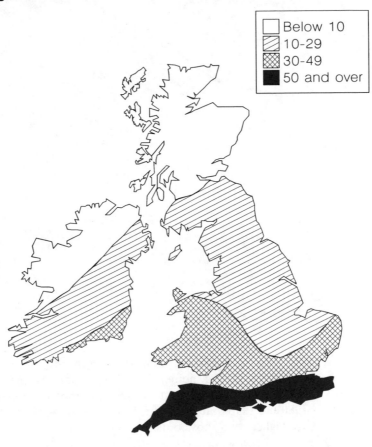

Legend:
- ☐ Below 10
- ▨ 10-29
- ▩ 30-49
- ■ 50 and over

Source: DH 1991

pain on deep inspiration, nausea and headache. At higher concentrations it impairs lung function. Sensitivity varies between individuals and also depends on length of exposure and level of exertion. It is not clear whether children with asthma are particularly sensitive to the effects of ozone itself. However, it makes them more sensitive to other pollutants that may be present, such as sulphur dioxide, and also more prone to exercise-induced attacks of asthma. The long-term effects of exposure to ozone are not known, but there is some evidence that high concentrations can cause permanent structural damage to the lungs.

There are no EC controls on ozone concentration. World Health Organisation guidelines recommend a maximum hourly average concentration of 75–100 parts per billion (p.p.b.) in the air. There is a marked north–south gradient in the number of hours exceeding these guidelines.

135

4.27 Trend in carbon monoxide emissions: source, United Kingdom 1980–90

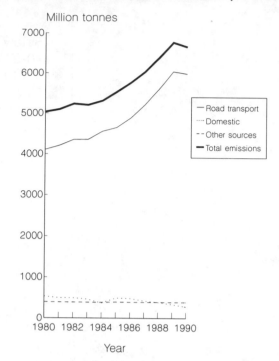

Million tonnes

Legend:
— Road transport
···· Domestic
-- Other sources
▬ Total emissions

Year

Source: DoE 1992

The effects of carbon monoxide on health have been described above (Pollution in the home). Road transport is the main outside source, accounting for 90 percent of carbon monoxide emissions in 1990. Between 1980 and 1990 road traffic emissions rose by 46 percent. Levels inside vehicles are higher than those outside.

Chronic exposure to lead impairs the mental development of young children (see Indoor air quality). One of the main sources of lead in the air is petrol. Others include coal combustion and metal works. Lead settles on the soil and water, so that children not only inhale it but also swallow it. Unleaded petrol has been available in the United Kingdom since 1986, and a steep fall in lead emissions from road transport has followed, despite a continuing increase in annual petrol consumption (which rose steadily from 16.13 million tonnes in 1975 to 24.31 million tonnes in 1990, a rise of 51 percent). There have been corresponding reductions in lead in dust and food and blood lead levels have been falling steadily since the mid-1970s (DoE 1990). A dramatic increase in sales followed the reduction in duty on unleaded petrol in April 1989, but by 1991 sales of unleaded petrol had risen only to 40 percent of total UK sales. Since October 1990 all new cars must be capable of running on unleaded petrol (CSO Social Trends 22).

4.28 Trend in lead emissions from petrol-engined road vehicles, United Kingdom 1975–90

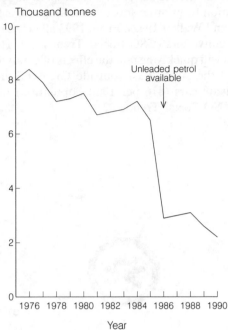

Thousand tonnes

Unleaded petrol available

Year

Source: DoE 1992

4.29 Projected trend in road traffic, Great Britain 1980–2025

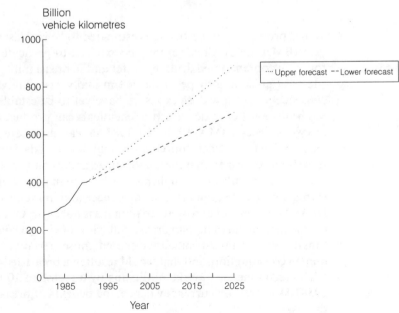

Billion vehicle kilometres

····· Upper forecast -- Lower forecast

Year

Source: DoT 1991

All motor traffic except two-wheelers

137

Traffic is the major source of air pollution. The amount of traffic, measured in terms of vehicle kilometres per year, is forecast to double by the year 2025. By contrast, pollution from other sources is falling and is forecast to continue to do so (Godlee and Walker 1992). From 1993 all new cars will have to be fitted with catalytic converters (CSO Social Trends 22). However, the projected increase in cars will quickly negate the effects of catalytic converters. In Great Britain in 1989 the South East (outside Greater London) had the highest number of private cars (416 per 1000 population) while Scotland had the lowest (281) (CSO Social Trends 22).

4.30   Chemical hazards

Many chemicals are known to be hazardous

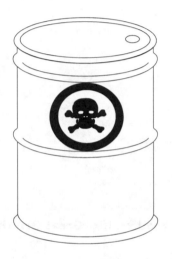

But their exact effects on health are still unknown

World production of pesticides is estimated to be increasing by 12.5 percent a year (BMA 1992). Children may be exposed to pesticide residues in treated foods, in contaminated drinking water and in breast milk. Although the acute effects of poisoning by pesticides are in many cases known, the longer-term consequences of low dose exposure have yet to be established (BMA 1992).

The disposal of toxic industrial chemicals can produce even more hazardous substances (BMA 1991). In 1985 it was discovered that soil around industrial waste incinerators contains high levels of dioxins and furans. It has since been confirmed that these substances are ubiquitous in the environment, with levels significantly higher in urban than in rural areas. Dioxin is extremely toxic to animals, causing cancer and immune system impairment. However, the extent of toxicity to humans is not clear. Of particular concern is the dioxin content of human breast milk. Surveys in the United Kingdom have found levels in breast milk that exceed those permitted in cow's milk for human consumption, and that would result in a breast-fed baby exceeding the WHO recommended intake of dioxins by a factor of 10 (Jensen 1983; Who 1988). However, on current evidence, the benefits of breast-feeding outweigh the risks.

Artificial radiation

Radiation causes cancer (Godlee and Walker 1992). Artificial sources account for around 13 percent of the annual average dose per person of 2.5 mSv of background radiation (see Figure 4.21). Children are not usually exposed to radiation from occupational sources. Similarly, if a child is not X-rayed it will not share the average 12 percent from medical imaging. About half of the contribution of nuclear fallout is due to the Chernobyl reactor accident and half to nuclear weapons fallout. Both of these components are decreasing.

For many children radiological medical procedures are the largest source of artificial exposure to radiation and there is much scope here for reduction. Every X-ray carries some risk, however small, of causing cancer.

Although discharges from nuclear power stations make up a tiny part of average background radiation, children living close by are exposed to higher levels. There is concern that these children have an increased risk of cancer. 'Clusters' of cases of childhood cancer have been found around nuclear power stations, particularly leukaemia in children under five. But they have also been found in areas with no nuclear installations or other potentially polluting sources. Such clusters suggest an environmental cause, but its nature remains to be established (OPCS 1991; Alberman 1992).

Beaches and bathing

Bathers in sewage-contaminated sea water are more likely than non-bathers to experience nausea, vomiting and diarrhoea, and they are at risk of respiratory, eye, throat and ear infections (Godlee and Walker 1992). In 1991, 24 percent of bathing waters in the UK failed to comply with EC standards for sewage contamination.

Pollution with global consequences

The ozone layer in the stratosphere shields the earth from ultraviolet light and plays a role in regulating the earth's temperature. Chlorofluorocarbons (CFCs) released into the atmosphere from aerosol sprays, refrigeration and light industry destroy stratospheric ozone (DoE 1992). Since the late 1980s there has been considerable thinning of the ozone over the poles in spring. There is evidence of a generalized thinning over the Northern Hemisphere of 4–5 percent in the past decade. The main effects on health are owing to increased exposure to ultraviolet-B radiation: increased risk of skin cancer, particularly malignant melanoma in the young, and 'snow blindness' and cataracts (Godlee and Walker 1992). The ecological consequences are potentially disastrous.

Certain gases trap outgoing radiation reflected back from the earth's surface, rather like the glass in a greenhouse. This has the effect of warming the lower atmosphere (the 'greenhouse effect'). The consequences are potentially catastrophic for all forms of life on the planet. Important 'greenhouse gases' are carbon dioxide (from power stations, industry and road transport), methane (from agriculture and waste disposal), nitrous oxide (from road transport) and CFCs (DoE 1992).

Discussion

The greatest threat to the young is a road traffic accident, and large numbers are killed and injured every day. Fear of traffic is a constant source of stress and anxiety. With an increasing number of cars, the roads have become more dangerous. Road accident figures, dramatic as they are, do not adequately reflect this because perception of the danger has led to restrictions on the freedom of children to use the streets (Hillman *et al.* 1990). Those in families with a car are ferried about in relative safety, those without are at risk as pedestrians. This is one of many inequalities that a society geared towards car-ownership creates. Cars also contribute to pollution, not just at a local level but also globally.

Although the home is regarded as a place of safety, many children are injured at home every day. The home may also be more polluted than outside, particularly when a parent smokes.

The prevention of accidents

Alongside the pain and personal costs suffered by injured children and their families are the enormous costs to society, measured not only in terms of cash for medical treatment or care of the disabled, but also in loss of human talent and potential. Much of this burden could be prevented. This is recognized in the Government's health strategy, 'The Health of the Nation', which selects accidental injury as a priority area. Explicit targets have been set: to reduce deaths from accidents among children aged under 15 by at least 33 percent, and among young people aged 15–24 by at least 25 percent, by 2005 (baseline 1990) (HoN 1992).

The physical environment is often the most obvious factor responsible for an accident, and prevention measures that build safeguards into the environment can be the most effective. The knowledge and technology exist to plan, build and engineer a safer environment for children: in the street (urban planning that separates pedestrians and cyclists from traffic; 'traffic calming' measures such as road humps) and elsewhere (soft surfaces in playgrounds). History provides ample evidence of how the design, manufacture and marketing of safer products leads to a decline in injuries. For example, regulations regarding flame-resistant children's nightdresses (1967) contrib- uted to a marked fall in burns (CAPT 1985); child-resistant containers and the packaging of medicines in small quantities have contributed to a decline in childhood poisoning over the past two decades (Jackson *et al.* 1983). Recommendations may need to be backed by legislation, for the builder and manufacturer, and also for all adults who determine the environment to which a child is exposed (for example, use of child restraints in cars). Legislation also needs to be enforced (speed limits are frequently breached with impunity).

The behaviour of the child or its guardian also determines whether or not an accident occurs. Education has a role to play in changing this behaviour. However, safety education has been disappointing (Pless and Arsenault 1987).

If the Government's targets are to be met, there needs to be coordination between Government Departments, with adequate resources devoted to tackling the injury problem. In many areas the action to reduce accidents is clear; for example, through traffic engineering. Adequate information systems to direct, monitor and evaluate preventive initiatives do not exist, and these should be set up. More research is needed, for example, to understand how best to address the death toll of teenagers on the roads or the striking gender difference in injuries.

Pollution control

The WHO guidelines for levels of air pollution are regularly exceeded in the United Kingdom. European Community directives are laxer than these. Even so, EC levels for sulphur dioxide and nitrogen dioxide are exceeded. There are no plans to introduce mandatory air quality standards, as in the Netherlands, Japan and the United States (FoE 1990a). There is a pressing need for international agreements to control air pollution since many pollutants, such as ozone and acid rain, do not respect national boundaries.

In the future it may be possible to reduce pollution from road traffic through technical advances. Meanwhile the use of cars should be discouraged, through, for example, financial disincentives, and alternatives, especially public transport, should be positively encouraged. Public opinion must be behind such measures, and there is a clear need to ensure maximum exposure to the message that traffic is a serious threat to health.

Medical imaging is an important source of radiation. Dose reduction is particularly important in children: their tissues are more radiosensitive than adults, they have longer for radiation-induced cancers to appear and infertility as a result of gonadal radiation is a serious complication (Dawood and Hall 1988). Unnecessary exposure must be avoided and gonadal shields correctly placed.

The risks of many other features of the physical environment, such as pesticides, hazardous wastes and nuclear fallout, may be perceived to be greater than they actually are. Often there is no good evidence that a particular pollutant is harmful or is not. More research is needed. In the light of this uncertainty, it would seem reasonable to suggest that the most vulnerable groups, including the unborn baby and the small child, be protected as far as possible.

Finally, the health not just of today's children but also of future generations depends on preserving the earth's fragile ecological balance. Unless urgent action is taken to prevent further thinning of the stratospheric ozone layer and global warming, we risk human and ecological catastrophe.

References

Publications other than routine data series

Alberman, E. (1992) 'After Windscale (Sellafield)' (Editorial), *British Medical Journal* 304: 1393–4.

Anonymous (1990) 'Asthma' (Editorial), *Journal of Epidemiology and Community Health* 44: 177–8.

Avery J. G. and Gibbs, B. (1985) 'Longterm disability following accidents in childhood', in *Proceedings of Symposium on Accidents in Childhood, 27–39*, Occasional Paper 7. London, Child Accident Prevention Trust.

British Medical Association (BMA) (1991) *Hazardous Waste and Human Health*. Oxford, Oxford University Press.

British Medical Association (BMA) (1992) *Pesticides, Chemicals and Health*. London, Edward Arnold.

BMJ (1992) 'Headlines', *British Medical Journal* 305: 668.

Burger, C. (1984) *Analysis of Child Poisoning Accidents*. London, DTI.

Child Accident Prevention Trust (CAPT) (1985) *Burn and Scald Accidents to Children*. London, Bedford Square Press/NCVO.

Child Accident Prevention Trust (CAPT) (1991) *Safe as Houses? Guidelines for the Safety of Children in Temporary Accommodation*. London, CAPT.

Committee on Environmental Hazards/Committee on Accident and Poison Prevention (CEH/CAPP), American Academy of Paediatrics (1987) 'Statement on childhood lead poisoning', *Pediatrics* 79: 457–65.

Craft, A. W. (1983) 'Circumstances surrounding death from accidental poisoning 1974–80', *Archives of Disease in Childhood* 58: 544–6.

Dawood, R. and Hall, C. M. (1988) 'Too much radiation for too many children?' (Editorial), *British Medical Journal* 296: 1277–8.

Department of the Environment (DoE) (1990) *UK Blood Lead Monitoring Programme 1984–87. Results for 1987*. Pollution report No. 28. London, HMSO.

Department of the Environment (DoE) (1992) *Digest of Environmental Protection and Water Statistics, No. 14*. London, DoE.

Department of Health (DoH) (1991) *Ozone*. First report of the Advisory Group on the Medical Aspects of Air Pollution Episodes. London, HMSO.

Department of Trade and Industry (DTI) (1990) *Home and Leisure Accident Report. Playgrounds*. London, DTI.

Department of Trade and Industry (DTI) (1992) *Home and Leisure Accident Report. Educational Institutions*. London, DTI.

Department of Transport (DoT) (1991) *Transport Statistics, Great Britain 1991*. London, HMSO.

Department of Transport (DoT) (1992) *Accident Fact Sheet No. 5*. London, DoT.

Faculty of Public Health Medicine (FPHM) (1992) *Committee on Health Promotion Guidelines for Health Promotion No. 30, Drinking Water*. London, FPHM.

Friends of the Earth (FoE) (1990a) 'Air quality', Briefing sheet. London, FoE.

Friends of the Earth (FoE) (1990b) 'Lead in drinking water', Briefing sheet. London, FoE.

Friends of the Earth (FoE) (1992) Press release, 28 September.

Godlee, F. and Walker, A. (1992) *Health and the Environment*. London, BMJ.

Health of the Nation (HoN) (1992) *A Strategy for Health in England*. London, HMSO.

Hillman, M., Adams, J. and Whitelegg, J. (1990) *One False Move . . . A Study of Children's Independent Mobility*. London, PSI Publishing.

Home Office (1992) *Home Office Fire Statistics UK 1990*. London, HMSO.

Jackson, R. H., Craft, A. W., Lawson, G. R., Beattie, A. B. and Sibert, J. R. (1983) Letter, *British Medical Journal* 287: 1468.

Jensen, A. A. (1983) 'Chemical contaminants in human milk', *Residue Reviews* 89: 1–127.

Kemp, A. and Sibert, J. R. (1992) 'Drowning and near drowning in children in the United Kingdom: lessons for prevention', *British Medical Journal* 304: 1143–6.

Lader, D. and Matheson, J. (1991) *Smoking among Secondary School Children in 1990*. London, HMSO.

Lowry, S. (1991) *Housing and Health*. London, BMJ.

McKeown, T. (1979) *The Role of Medicine*. Oxford: Basil Blackwell.

Mihill, C. and Linton, M. (1992) 'Four million children at passive smoking risk', *Guardian* 13 October.

Ministry of Agriculture, Fisheries and Food (MAFF) (1989) *Lead in Food: Progress Report*. Food Surveillance Paper No. 27. London, HMSO.

National Radiological Protection Board (NRPB) (1992) *Radon in Dwellings in England*. London, HMSO.

O'Neill, P. (1992) 'Lead paint: still a threat to children', *British Medical Journal* 305: 440.

OPCS (1991) *The Geographical Epidemiology of Childhood Leukaemia and Non-Hodgkin's Lymphomas in Great Britain 1966–83*. Studies in medical and population subjects No. 53. London, HMSO.

Pless, I. B. and Arsenault, L. (1987) 'The role of health education in the prevention of injuries to children', *Journal of Social Issues* 43: 87–103.

Read, C. (1991) *Air Pollution and Child Health*. London, Greenpeace.

Royal College of Physicians (RCP) (1992) *Smoking and the Young*. London, RCP.

Strachan, D. P. (1992) 'Causes and control of chronic respiratory disease: looking beyond the smokescreen' (Editorial), *Journal of Epidemiology and Community Health* 46: 177–9.

Who (1988) *Assessment of Health Risks in Infants Associated with Exposure to PCBs, PCDDs and PCDFs in Breast Milk*. Environmental Health Series No. 29. Copenhagen, WHO.

Routine data series

Office of Population Censuses and Surveys:
  OPCS MB4 Hospital Inpatient Enquiry
  OPCS DH2 Mortality Statistics: Cause
  OPCS DH4 Mortality Statistics: Accidents and Violence
  OPCS General Household Survey
Central Statistical Office:
  CSO Social Trends
Registrar General for Northern Ireland:
  RG N Ireland Annual Reports
Registrar General for Scotland:
  RG Scotland Annual Reports

CHAPTER 5 Cultural environment

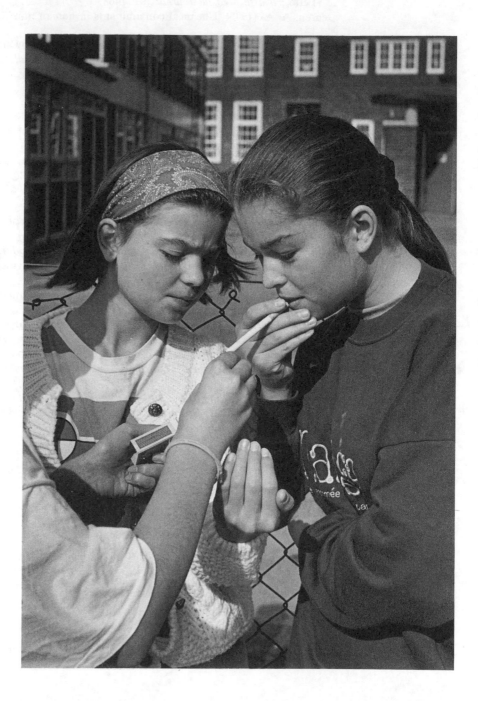

Key facts

- Only 2 percent of couples are knowingly risking unplanned parenthood.

- A quarter of 15 year olds and a third of 16–19 year olds smoke. Smoking is increasing among young women and not declining among young men.

- Most adult smokers started smoking as adolescents.

- Although there has been a decrease in alcohol-related road accidents, in 1990 a fifth of drivers killed had alcohol levels over the legal limit.

- Thirty percent of fathers with a child under five drink heavily.

- 'Hard' drugs have been offered to 15–18 percent of 15 year olds; 3–7 percent report having used them.

- Deaths from volatile substance abuse are increasing rapidly among teenagers.

- Boys aged 11–16 exercise twice as often as girls.

- Only two-thirds of infants are breast-fed at birth and only a fifth at six months old.

Introduction

This chapter describes the influences on child health traditionally described as behaviour or lifestyle. Individuals are often thought to have more control over these factors than over their socioeconomic or physical environment. The topics covered, which may have a positive or negative impact on health, are planning parenthood, smoking, drinking, drugs, exercise and diet. Some is adult behaviour (planning parenthood, drunken driving). Other behaviour is by children and teenagers themselves (drugs, exercise).

Values, habits and attitudes to health are shaped by gender roles, social and ethnic origins, education, family and peer group pressures, exposure to the media and other influences. Health behaviour, therefore, cannot be separated from the social and cultural environment; it is important to consider these topics in context rather than as solely the responsibility of the individual. This has important implications for prevention.

Behaviour is difficult to measure and reliance is usually placed on individuals' reports. This may result in an underestimation of the problem, since many of the areas covered, such as drinking and drug-taking, are very sensitive. There are still considerable gaps in our knowledge.

Patterns of behaviour in young people are particularly important as they set the scene for healthy or unhealthy lifestyles in adult life.

Planning parenthood

Planned parenthood is a major determinant of child health (RCOG 1991). The prevention of unwanted births was probably the most important factor in the reduction of infant and child mortality from non-infectious conditions over the last century (McKeown 1976).

5.1 Women risking unplanned pregnancy*, Great Britain 1991

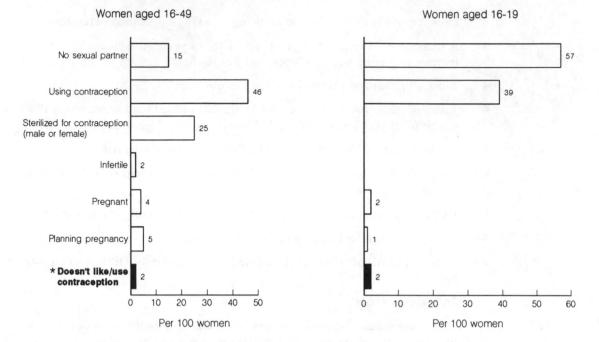

Women aged 16-49

	Per 100 women
No sexual partner	15
Using contraception	46
Sterilized for contraception (male or female)	25
Infertile	2
Pregnant	4
Planning pregnancy	5
* Doesn't like/use contraception	2

Women aged 16-19

	Per 100 women
No sexual partner	57
Using contraception	39
Pregnant	2
Planning pregnancy	1
* Doesn't like/use contraception	2

Source: OPCS GHS, personal communication

The use of contraception has become widespread in Great Britain. Only 2 percent of women aged 16–49 say they are taking no precautions despite being at risk of an unplanned pregnancy (OPCS GHS, personal communication).

Sterilization is increasingly popular and is now the contraceptive method used by 25 percent of couples (OPCS GHS, personal communication). However, free sterilization is not available as a form of family planning to the residents of at least 17 Districts (out of 200), and in some others free operations are available only for couples on low incomes (Ewart 1991).

The contribution of abortion to reducing the potential number of unwanted births is substantial. Twenty percent of all pregnant women (excluding pregnancies ending in miscarriage) decide to abort their pregnancy. Fewer than 1 percent of abortions are due to fetal abnormality.

The proportion of conceptions ending in abortion increased from 14 percent in 1972, the first year in which the transfer between illegal and legal abortions following the Abortion Act 1967 was probably complete (Botting 1991). Data are not published in this form for Scotland, and abortion is not legal in Northern Ireland.

146

5.2 Conceptions ending in maternity or abortion: age, England and Wales 1989

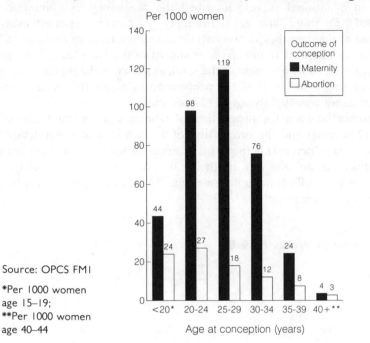

Per 1000 women

Outcome of
conception
■ Maternity
□ Abortion

Source: OPCS FM1

*Per 1000 women
age 15–19;
**Per 1000 women
age 40–44

Age at conception (years)

5.3 Births following unintended pregnancy: age of mother, England and Wales 1989

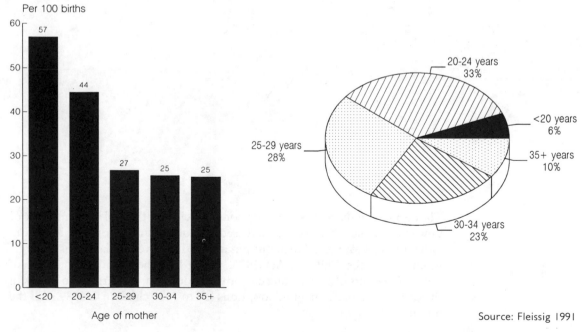

Per 100 births

Age of mother

20-24 years
33%

<20 years
6%

35+ years
10%

30-34 years
23%

25-29 years
28%

Source: Fleissig 1991

147

Despite widespread use of contraception, 31 percent of mothers of six month old babies in a national survey described the pregnancy as unintended (Fleissig 1991). Of those who gave this reply, 70 percent reported using contraception at the time they conceived. Over half the teenage mothers (57 percent) had not intended to conceive, as shown in the bar chart. Teenage mothers contributed only 6 percent of the total, as shown in the pie chart. In a similar survey conducted in 1984 the proportion of births following unintended pregnancies was slightly lower (27 percent).

The difference between the proportion of women risking unintentional pregnancy (2 percent) and the proportion of women in whom unintended pregnancy occurs (4 percent) is in part explained by the difference between reported behaviour on one day in the year and the risk of conceiving throughout the year. All contraceptive methods have failure rates, even when used correctly and consistently.

5.4 Trend in adoptions, England and Wales 1959–89

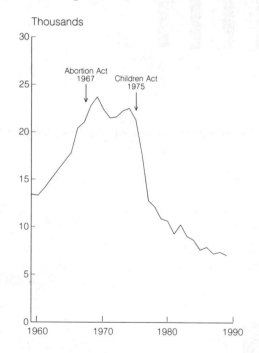

Source: OPCS FM2

The decrease in the number of adoptions coincides with a fall in the number of unwanted babies, because of increased use of contraception and abortion. Other reasons for the fall in adoptions are the improved social status of single mothers and the Children Act 1975, which had the effect for children of divorced parents of substituting custody for adoption. After rising to a peak in the early 1970s the number of adoptions fell to 7000 children in 1989, half the number adopted in 1959.

The average age of children at adoption has increased gradually, although infants remain more likely than older children to be adopted. In 1989 in England and Wales 16 per 10,000 infants were adopted. Adoptions followed a similar trend in Scotland, falling from 2300 in 1969 to 800 in 1990 (RG Scotland 1991).

5.5 Teenage parents: age, England and Wales 1990

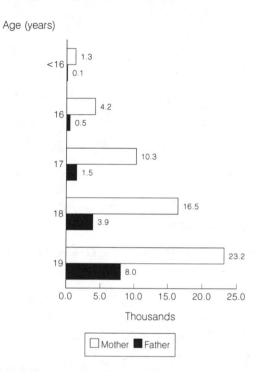

Age (years)

Source: OPCS FM1

In England and Wales in 1990 there were 55,500 births to mothers under 20, of which 42 percent were to 19 year olds and 2 percent (1300) were to under 16s. The number of young men known to have become fathers under 20 years old was 13,900, of whom 18 percent were married.

The teenage birth rate fell from 30.4 per 1000 women aged 15–19 in 1980 to 26.9 in 1983 before rising to 33.2 in 1991 (England and Wales). In Scotland the rate also fell until the mid-1980s before increasing to 31.9 per 1000 in 1990, a similar level to England and Wales. The rate in Northern Ireland in 1990 was slightly lower at 29.3 per 1000 (CSO AAS 128).

149

5.6 Trend in teenage birth rate, England and Wales 1961–91

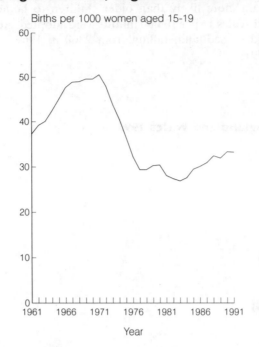

Births per 1000 women aged 15-19

Source: OPCS FMI,
Population Trends

Year

Teenage abortion

5.7 Trend in abortions to women age 16–19 years, Great Britain 1970–91

Per 1000 women

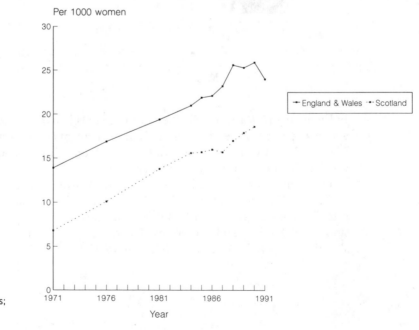

England & Wales · Scotland

Source: OPCS
Population Trends;
CSA 1991

Year

150

A pregnancy that is unwanted and distressing to the extent that the woman decides to seek an abortion is a common form of acute morbidity among teenagers. In 1991 in England and Wales, 24 per 1000 women aged 16–19 and 6 per 1000 aged 14–15 had an abortion (OPCS Population Trends). In Scotland the rate for age 16–19 years was 19 per 1000 in 1990 (CSA 1991). Young women in Northern Ireland, where the law has not yet been liberalized, must go abroad to obtain a legal abortion. In the years 1988–90 an annual average of 484 teenagers from Northern Ireland are known to have had an abortion in England and Wales, 18 of them under 16 years of age (OPCS AB 15–17).

5.8 **Teenage conceptions ending in maternity or abortion: age, England and Wales 1990**

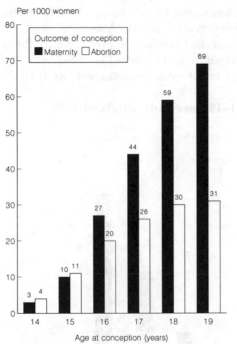

Per 1000 women

Outcome of conception
■ Maternity □ Abortion

Age at conception (years)

Source: OPCS FM1/20

The younger the teenager, the more likely a pregnancy is to be aborted. Over half of pregnant 14–15 year olds choose abortion, whereas 69 percent of pregnant women aged 19 at conception continue with their pregnancy. Miscarriages are not included in these data.

Complications of abortion increase the later an abortion is performed. Younger women are at increased risk of having late abortions, being less likely to recognize the pregnancy early, less aware of the urgency and less able to avoid delays in NHS referral (Alberman and Dennis 1984). The proportion of abortions performed at or after 13 weeks' gestation was 22 percent for girls under 16 years, 18 percent for young women aged 16–19 years and 11 percent at age 20 and over, in 1988 (OPCS AB 17).

One reason for delay is the difficulty of obtaining free treatment in the NHS for this form of acute hospital care. In 1990, 17,700 teenagers, or 46 percent of the total having abortions, had to pay for the operation in the private sector, many having tried to obtain NHS treatment in time.

Smoking

> Tobacco is the most dangerous consumer product the world has ever known.
> Royal College of Physicians 1992

The harmful effects of active smoking are undisputed. A quarter of 15 year olds and a third of 18 year olds are smokers, and smoking is increasing among young women. Smoking during adolescence has an immediate effect on health, increasing respiratory disease and reducing physical fitness. It also has long-term effects on adult health. Almost all adult smokers became addicted as teenagers, and the harmful effects of tobacco, for example the risk of lung cancer, are related to the number of years an individual has smoked over and above the amount of tobacco consumed (RCP 1992).

5.9   Regular smoking among 11–15 year olds, England 1990

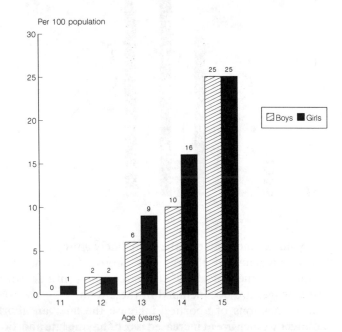

Source: Lader and Matheson 1991

A quarter of 15 year olds regularly smoke at least one cigarette a week. The average for boys who smoke is 56 cigarettes a week and for girls 49. Only a third of 15 year olds have never smoked (Lader and Matheson 1991). Similar results were obtained in a survey in Northern Ireland (Northern Ireland DHSS 1991).

Under the Protection of Children (Tobacco) Act 1986, it is illegal to sell tobacco to anyone below the age of 16. Despite this, only 15 percent of children were refused cigarettes the last time they tried to buy them, and approximately 17 million cigarettes a week are consumed by children aged 11–15 in England, 0.8 million in Wales and 1.5 million in Scotland (Lader and Matheson 1991). The illegal market of sales to under 16s is estimated to be worth £100 million a year (ASH 1992). In an attempt to reduce sales to children the Children and Young Persons (Protection from Tobacco) Act which came into force on 1 March 1992 banned the sale of single cigarettes and imposed tougher fines on shopkeepers who sell cigarettes to children (*BMJ* 1992).

5.10 Regular smokers among 11–15 year olds: smokers in the family, England 1990

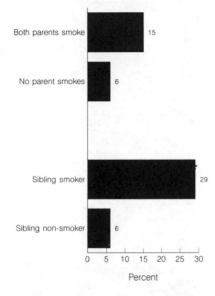

Source: Lader and
Matheson 1991

Parents who smoke jeopardize their children's health by exposing them to passive smoking (see Chapter 4). They also influence their children's smoking behaviour. Children whose parents both smoke are more than twice as likely to smoke themselves as children of non-smoking parents (15 percent compared to 6 percent). A third of married parents living with dependent children are smokers (OPCS GHS 21).

Siblings also affect smoking behaviour. Of children with a brother or sister who smoked, 29 percent are regular smokers themselves compared with only 6 percent of children with non-smoking siblings (Lader and Matheson 1991).

A longitudinal study of factors associated with secondary schoolchildren in England beginning to smoke identified female gender, siblings smoking, parents smoking, living in a lone parent family and low educational aspirations (Goddard 1990). A survey of secondary schoolchildren in Wales (where smoking rates are among the highest in Europe) found pupils are more likely to smoke if their parents smoke or have a permissive attitude to smoking, if their best friend is a smoker, or if they feel alienated or under-achieve at school (Smith 1991).

5.11   Trends in smoking: age, Great Britain 1972–90

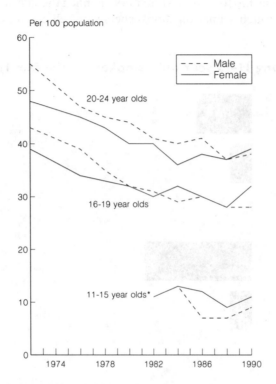

Per 100 population

Source: OPCS GHS 21;
Lader and Matheson
1991

*England only

Smoking has declined less among 16–19 year olds and 20–24 year olds than in the population as a whole. Between 1972 and 1990 the prevalence of cigarette smoking among all ages over 16 fell by 35 percent (40 percent for men and 29 percent for women), but among 16–19 year olds the reduction was only 27 percent (35 percent for men and 18 percent for women). Indeed the decline among young people has levelled off in recent years, and smoking even seems to be on the increase among young women. Targeting of women, specifically young women, by the tobacco industry led to a steady increase in cigarette advertising expenditure in women's magazines to £9.7 million by 1988 (Amos *et al.* 1991).

   The average weekly cigarette consumption for smokers aged 16–19 is 89 for men and 80 for women, compared to 110 and 92 per week for smokers aged 20–24.

154

5.12 Smokers aged 16–19: socioeconomic group of 'head of household', Great Britain 1990

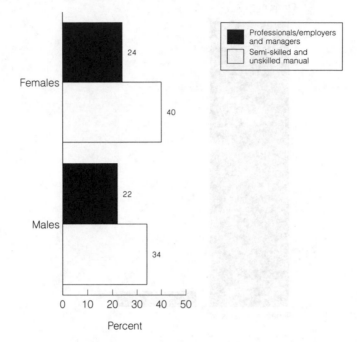

Source: E. Goddard, personal communication

Young people from households headed by semi-skilled and unskilled manual workers are more likely to smoke than those from professional and managerial households, according to unpublished estimates from the General Household Survey.

5.13 Adult smokers: age began regular smoking, Great Britain 1988

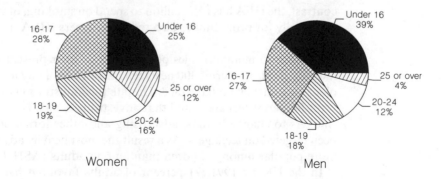

Source: OPCS GHS

Most adult smokers start smoking as adolescents. Of all current and ex-regular smokers aged 16 or over, a quarter of women and two-fifths of men started smoking before they were 16 while more than 70 percent of both sexes started before they were 20.

5.14 Expenditure on publicity for and against smoking, England and Wales 1992

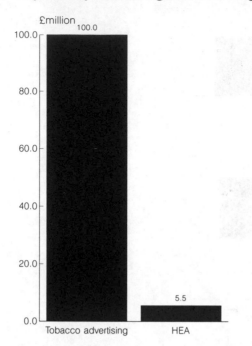

£million

Source: ASH 1992;
Health Education
Authority, personal
communication

The Royal College of Physicians has called on the government to use the two most effective means it has to reduce smoking among young people – banning tobacco advertising and raising the price of cigarettes (RCP 1992).

Government funding of anti-smoking education through the Health Education Authority (HEA) is dwarfed by the amount spent by the tobacco industry on advertising. The estimate for the industry is £100 million a year, £87 million on advertising and the remainder on sponsorship (ASH 1992). In contrast, the HEA has £5.5 million to spend on smoking, of which £2 million is specifically for programmes directed to teenagers (HEA, personal communication).

In order to maintain sales of cigarettes at their present level the tobacco industry needs to recruit 300 new teenage smokers a day in the UK to replace older customers who have died. Despite the industry's claim that it does not want to recruit teenagers and that advertising is merely to persuade existing smokers to change brands, advertising and other forms of promotion have been targeted on teenagers. As a result the most heavily advertised brands are more popular among children than among adults (ASH 1992).

In the UK by 1991, 71 percent of adults favoured banning all cigarette advertising. Advertising has been banned in France, Italy, Portugal, Norway, Finland, Iceland, Canada, Australia and New Zealand (ASH 1992).

Price is one of the most important factors affecting cigarette consumption, particularly among young people starting to smoke, and cigarettes are relatively cheap. In 1991 a cigarette cost on average only 10p compared to

35–50p for a soft drink. The UK income from tobacco tax was £6000 million in 1988–9 (House of Commons Hansard 1990a). It has been argued that the government is reluctant to increase the price and lose this tax revenue. The relationship of consumption to price is such, however, that a 1 percent rise in price will cause a fall in consumption of only 0.5 percent (RCP 1992). The main argument against increased taxation is that the tax is regressive, falling most heavily on smokers with low incomes.

Drinking

Irresponsible drinking puts children at risk by contributing to family violence, child neglect and abuse, traffic accidents, and accidents and fires in the home (Anderson 1991; Secretary of State for Health 1991). Drinking behaviour of adults that jeopardizes the health of children and teenagers, and the drinking behaviour of teenagers themselves are described.

5.15 Trend in percentage of 16–19 year old drivers killed having excess blood alcohol*, Great Britain 1979–90

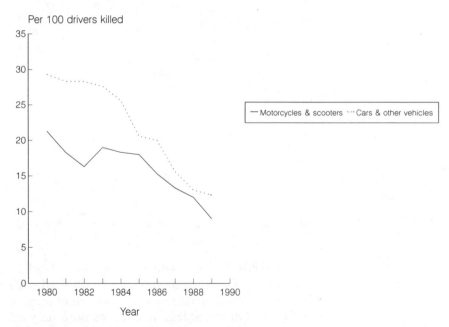

Source: DoT 1991

*More than 80 mg per 100 ml blood

Three year averages

An extreme measure of the amount of drinking and driving is the number of drivers killed in accidents when their blood alcohol level was over the legal limit. This gives only a partial indication of the impact of drunken driving on child health, omitting casualties caused to pedestrians, passengers and occupants of other cars. The child pedestrian casualty rate in the UK is one of the highest in Europe (see Chapter 4).

In 1989 a tenth of teenage drivers killed on the roads and a fifth of drivers of all ages killed had alcohol levels over 80 mg per 100 ml of blood. The proportion was twice as high among 20–29 year olds as among 16–19 year olds. There has been a reduction in the proportion of alcohol-related deaths in the last decade, which may reflect a true decrease in drunken driving or only a fall in the proportion of accidents that are fatal to the driver without a reduction in casualties among passengers and pedestrians.

5.16 Driving after drinking over the 'safe' limit*: age and sex, England and Wales 1987 and 1989

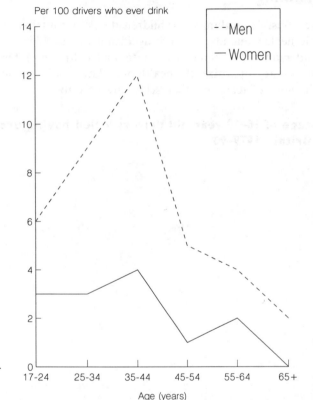

Source: Goddard 1991

*Five units or more for men, four or more for women

Another method of estimating the amount of drinking and driving is by sample survey. Of all drivers aged over 16 who had a drink in the last week and who held a current driving licence, 7 percent of men and 3 percent of women said they had driven at least once in the previous week when over the 'safe' limit. The survey defined five units or more for men and four units or more for women as the amount at which the legal limit was likely to be exceeded. A unit is a glass of wine or half a pint of beer. Among the group aged 35–44, 12 percent had done so. These are likely to be underestimates.

Driving over the safe alcohol limit may have decreased. Among men over 16 who had a drink in the last week and who held a current driving licence, the proportion who reported that they had ever driven in the last year over the legal limit decreased from 22 percent in 1987 to 15 percent in 1989. There was an increase, however, in the number of drivers in the population (see Chapter 4).

In July 1992 the maximum prison sentence for causing death by careless driving while under the influence of alcohol was increased from six months to five years, with disqualification from driving for at least two years.

5.17 Parents' heavy drinking* in last week: age of youngest child, England and Wales 1987 and 1989

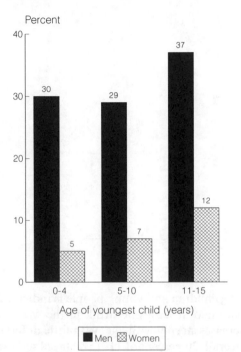

Percent

Age of youngest child (years)

■ Men ▨ Women

Source: Goddard 1991

*More than 21 units for men, 14 for women

Heavy drinking by parents can affect the quality of life and health of children in many ways. An OPCS survey (Goddard 1991) found that, although parents drink less than non-parents, 30 percent of married men living with a child under five drank heavily (defined as over 21 units for men, 14 for women) in the previous week. In contrast to smoking, the older the child the more likely the father was to drink this amount. Some children had fathers with 'very high' consumption, defined as 51 units per week. Unfortunately these data were limited to married men.

The proportion of mothers drinking heavily was lower than fathers at all ages of children. By the time the youngest child was aged 11–15, 12 percent of mothers reported drinking more than 14 units per week. Drinking levels were similar among mothers living on their own with children. Similar patterns were found for Great Britain in the GHS for 1990–1 (OPCS GHS 21).

159

5.18   Young people who had a drink in last week: age 11–15 years, England 1990; 16–24 years, England and Wales 1989

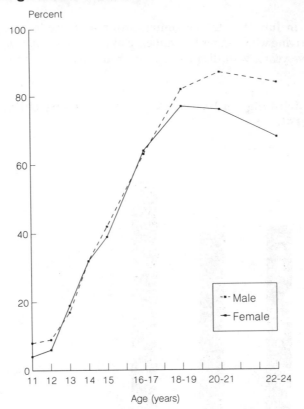

Percent

Age (years)

Source: Lader and
Matheson 1991;
Goddard 1991

Drinking among children and young people is indicated by survey reports of the number who had at least one drink in the week before interview. This proportion increases steeply with age, with little difference between the sexes until 18–19. Overall, 20 percent of 11–15 year old girls and 22 percent of boys had a drink in the last week; girls drank on average 2.7 units in the week and boys 5.7. The rate for both sexes declines from age 20.

Among those who drank in the last week, heavy drinking was more common among 18–24 year olds than other age groups, and among men than women. More than twice as many men as women of all ages combined drank heavily, 26 percent compared to 10 percent. It is particularly worrying that 13 percent of young men and 7 percent of young women aged 16–17 who drank at all were heavy drinkers according to the standards for adults.

At all ages women in manual socioeconomic groups who drink at all are more likely to drink heavily. The difference between socioeconomic groups is smaller for men (OPCS GHS 21).

5.19 Heavy drinking* in last week: age and sex, Great Britain 1988

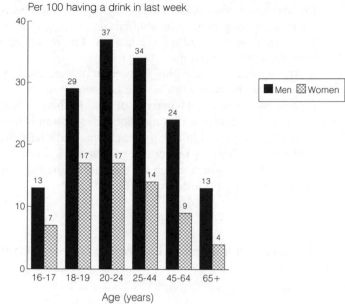

Per 100 having a drink in last week

■ Men ☒ Women

Age (years)

Source: OPCS GHS

*More than 21 units
for men, 14 for women

5.20 'Binge' drinking* in last week: age and sex, England and Wales 1989

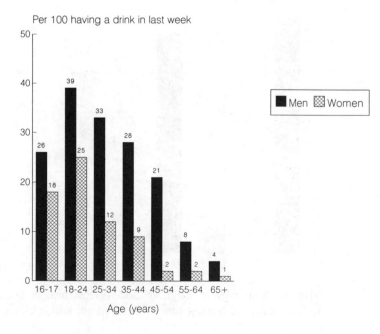

Per 100 having a drink in last week

■ Men ☒ Women

Age (years)

Source: Goddard 1991

*More than eight units
for men, six for
women,
on one occasion

161

'Binge' drinking may pose an even greater risk of accidents and violence to children and teenagers. This is defined as more than eight units for men and six for women on one occasion. Like heavy drinking, 'binge' drinking was more common among men than women at all ages, and more common among 18–24 year olds than other age groups. The reduction with age was steeper than for heavy drinking.

Among all 18–24 year olds, 33 percent of men and 18 percent of women had at least one 'binge session' in the last week. Among all 16–17 year olds 16 percent of males and 11 percent of females had a 'binge session'.

There is no evidence that alcohol consumption is increasing among young people aged under 24 following the change in the licensing laws and even some evidence that drinking fell among men aged 18–24 between the late 1970s and the late 1980s. Young women are the only women among whom consumption has not increased (Goddard 1991).

5.21 Fifteen year olds who had a drink in last week: country, United Kingdom 1990

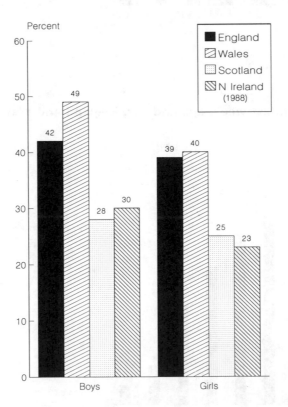

Source: Lader and
Matheson 1991

More 15 year olds in England and Wales than in Scotland and Northern Ireland reported having one or more alcoholic drinks in the previous week.

162

Drugs

5.22   Drug use by 15–16 year olds: type of drug, Wales 1990

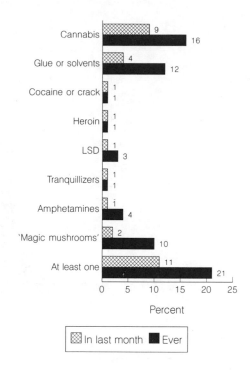

Source: Smith and
Nutbeam 1992

In a survey of Welsh 15–16 year olds, 11 percent had used at least one of the listed drugs or substances in the last month and 21 percent ever. There was no difference between manual and non-manual families or between boys and girls.

In a survey of 15 year olds in England and Wales, 15 percent of girls and 18 percent of boys had been offered at least one of LSD, heroin, ecstasy, cocaine or crack ('hard' drugs), while 19 percent of girls and 20 percent of boys had been offered at least one of cannabis, amphetamines or tranquillizers ('soft' drugs). Solvents had been offered to 9 percent of both girls and boys. A higher proportion of children in London and the South East had been exposed to drugs than elsewhere in England and Wales. White children and those in higher socioeconomic groups were slightly more likely to have been offered drugs. Only 7 percent of boys and 3 percent of girls had used a 'hard' drug, 18 percent of boys and 14 percent of girls had used a 'soft' drug, and 4 percent of boys and 2 percent of girls had used solvents. Use of drugs, as opposed to exposure, was higher in the lower socioeconomic groups (HEA 1992).

5.23   Trend in deaths from volatile substance abuse, age 9–20 years, United Kingdom 1981–90

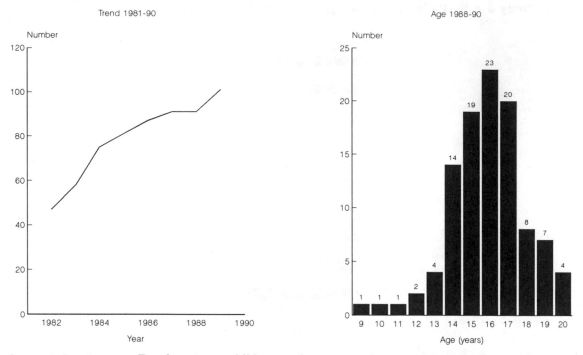

Trend 1981-90

Number

Year

Age 1988-90

Number

Age (years)

Source: A. Esmail,
personal
communication
1992

Three year averages

Deaths among children and teenagers from volatile substance abuse rose steeply in the last decade. As the Home Office statistics are known to underestimate drug-related deaths, data collected by St George's Hospital, London, have been used. In the three years 1988–90 there was an average of 23 deaths a year among 16 year olds.

The volatile substances commonly inhaled or sniffed include glue, aerosols (air freshener, deodorants, hair lacquer), nail varnish remover, fire extinguishers, cigarette lighter refills and typewriter correcting fluid. Following the Intoxicating Substances (Supply) Act 1985, which made it an offence to supply intoxicating substances to children under 18 if there is reason to believe they will be used to achieve intoxication, there was a transfer of deaths from glue and solvents to cigarette lighter refills and aerosols. As these new substances may be more lethal, nearly a third of the resulting deaths are now the result of the teenager's first experiment (Esmail *et al.* 1992).

Doctors are required to notify the Home Office of anyone addicted to one of the controlled drugs (all opiates apart from cocaine). However, as drug misuse is a largely clandestine activity, an unknown proportion of addicts appears in the Home Office statistics. Young people under 21 make up 17 percent of all new notifications, twice as many men as women.

Apparent time-trends in notification are the result of changes in treatment policy as well as changes in addiction. In every age group the number of newly notified addicts peaked in 1985 (Home Office 1991).

Exercise

The main contribution of regular exercise in childhood is to long-term health, partly through establishing an active lifestyle (*Lancet* 1992). Unfortunately there have been only a few studies of exercise in childhood, and no national data are available on long-term trends. The increased use of cars is likely to have led to a substantial reduction in exercise, for example in journeys to school. Between 1981 and 1990 the distance travelled by people of all ages in cars increased by 39 percent in Great Britain (CSO Social Trends 22).

5.24 Trend in physical activity outside of school, age 11–16 years, four or more hours per week, Wales 1986 and 1988

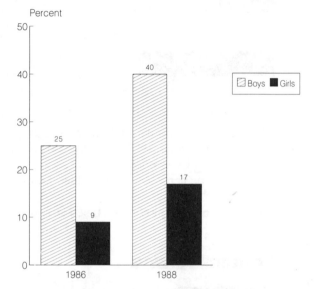

Source: Nutbeam 1989

The most striking fact about exercise among 11–16 year olds is the gender difference, boys being almost twice as active as girls (Nutbeam 1989; Riddoch *et al.* 1991). There is some evidence in recent years that participation in active sports is increasing overall, and at the same time the gender gap seems to be closing (Sports Council 1990). However, there is concern that physical education (PE) in schools has declined since 1985 as a direct result of changes in the educational system. In 1990, 71 percent of children under 14 in state schools had less than two hours PE a week (Scottish Sports Council 1989; Secondary Heads Association 1990).

Physical activity outside of school, defined as 'games or sport that make you out of breath', was surveyed among Welsh schoolchildren in 1986 and 1988. Boys were more active than girls. In both groups activity increased between 1986 and 1988 (Nutbeam 1989).

In Northern Ireland more than twice as many boys as girls aged 11–18 take physical exercise. Teenagers aged 17 and 18 are half as active as 11–14 year olds (Riddoch *et al.* 1991).

5.25 Exercise, age 16–24 years, England 1990

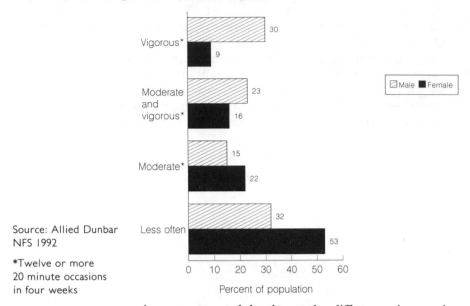

Source: Allied Dunbar
NFS 1992

*Twelve or more
20 minute occasions
in four weeks

Among young adults the gender differences in exercise persist. A survey of 16–24 year olds in England in 1990 found that 30 percent of men participated in vigorous exercise on 12 or more 20 minute occasions in the last four weeks, compared to only 9 percent of women (Allied Dunbar NFS 1992).

5.26 Active sports, age 16–19 years, participation in last four weeks, Great Britain 1990

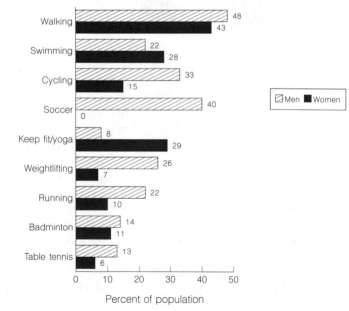

Source: OPCS GHS

Almost one-half of 16–19 year olds report having gone for a walk as a leisure activity in the last four weeks (the survey was conducted throughout 1990). The most popular active sport among young men is soccer, while keep-fit or yoga and swimming are most popular with young women. Ninety percent of young men and 75 percent of young women take part in some sport or leisure activity other than walking. The numbers taking exercise are unknown, however, as less active sports (darts, snooker, billiards and pool) are included (Matheson 1991). Walking, swimming, football and cycling are also the most popular active sports among this age group in Northern Ireland (Northern Ireland DHSS 1992).

Diet

An adequate and balanced diet is essential for children's growth and health. In addition, eating habits established in childhood tend to influence behaviour in adult life.

5.27   Trend in infants breast-fed: age, England and Wales 1975–90

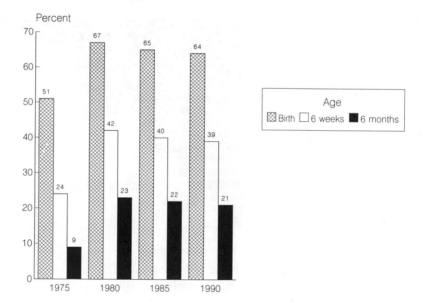

Source: DH 1988;
OPCS 1992

Breast milk provides the best nutrition for normal babies for at least the first 4–6 months of life (DH 1991), and affords beneficial effects such as protection against gastrointestinal and respiratory infections (Howie *et al.* 1990). In the early 1970s breast-feeding was at its lowest level, but following the Oppé Report (DHSS 1974) and changes in public and professional attitudes, the proportion of infants breast-fed at birth in England and Wales rose from 51 percent in 1975 to 67 percent in 1980. This rise has not continued (Emery *et al.* 1990; OPCS 1992).

167

Social and regional disparities in breast-feeding exist: more than four times as many infants are breast-fed at six weeks in social class I than in class V. Breast-feeding rates in Scotland are about three-quarters those in England and Wales (DH 1988).

Targets have been proposed to increase breast-feeding in England by the year 2000 to 75 percent at birth and 50 percent at six weeks (Secretary of State for Health 1991). The UK government supports the WHO 1981 International Code of Marketing of Breast-milk Substitutes and the Department of Health for England has asked Health Authorities to take measures to secure the aims of the code (DH Health Circular (89) 21). However, the market for baby milk grew in value in the UK by 21 percent in the year to October 1990 (Amery and Tomkins 1991). Since May 1991 the member governments of the EC have been allowed to prohibit advertising, and in July 1992 the Secretary of State promised legislation to implement the directive (Hansard 2 July 1992).

The 1992 EC directive on maternity leave and pay may increase breast-feeding by giving more women the right to paid maternity leave (Beecham 1992; Wolf 1992).

5.28   Percentage of children age 11–16 years eating various foods daily, Wales 1988

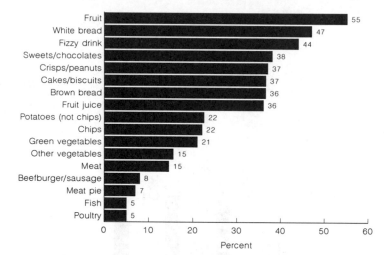

Source: Nutbeam 1989

Most children in the UK are adequately nourished, and in many, intakes of total dietary energy, protein and other nutrients are well in excess of healthy requirements.

Trends towards healthier eating habits, including less saturated fat and sugar, are reflected in a reduction over the last decade of average dietary energy intakes in most age groups (MAFF 1990). The Department of Health has recommended reductions in consumption of sucrose (packet sugar) to not more than 10 percent of dietary energy and fats to 35 percent (DH 1991). However, fatty and sweet foods, such as fizzy drinks, sweets, chocolates, crisps and chips, still make up a large part of the diet of school-age children (Golding et al. 1984; DH 1989; Nutbeam 1989).

Children's dietary patterns show class differences. Children in higher social classes have higher intakes of iron and vitamin C, and obtain more of these and of total energy from milk and healthy foods and less from chips and fizzy drinks (Golding *et al.* 1984; DH 1989). Because vitamin C assists iron absorption, a higher intake may protect against iron deficiency.

In the UK a greater proportion of Asian children are iron deficient, anaemic, deficient in vitamin D and at risk of rickets than white children of the same age (O'Hare *et al.* 1984; Ehrhardt 1986). Vitamin D deficiency occurs in 6 percent of Asian girls aged 13–15 years. While nutritional deficiencies are found in all disadvantaged groups, traditional diets contribute to this morbidity in some Asian children.

5.29 Trend in schoolchildren taking school meals, England 1973–90

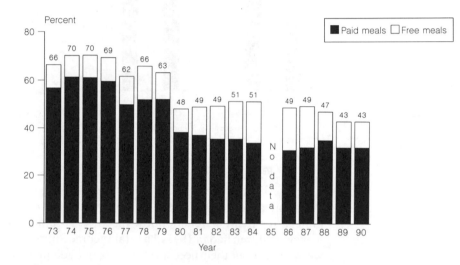

Source: DES 1979–90

The availability of school meals and possibly their nutritional value has declined in the last decade. The Education Act 1980 abolished nutritional standards which had been in force in various forms since 1955. The Act also ended the universal availability of school meals at fixed prices and restricted free meals to children of parents receiving Supplementary Benefit and Family Income Supplement (Berger 1990). As a result, many schoolchildren are eating 'unhealthy 'snack' foods for what is often the main meal of the day (National Dairy Council 1982; Food Commission 1991). This is especially so in lower income families.

The number of pupils in England taking school meals fell from some 4,600,000 (63 percent) in 1979 to 3,500,000 (48 percent) in 1980. The Social Security Act 1986 further reduced entitlement with effect from 1988, with free meals now being provided only for those in receipt of Income Support. In 1990, 32 percent of pupils took paid meals and 11 percent free meals (the reduction between 1988 and 1989 is due to a change in the method of calculation) (DES 1990).

169

5.30 Cost of adequate diet compared to Income Support*: family composition, United Kingdom 1991–2

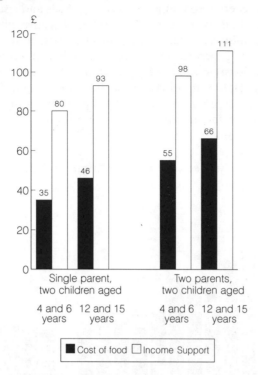

Source: Leather 1992

*Including Child Benefit

Providing an adequate diet – let alone a healthy one – for their children is difficult for many parents on low incomes. A family of two adults and two teenage children had in 1991–2 a total Income Support allowance of £110.95 a week to meet *all* their needs. A 'modest but adequate' diet would take up 59 percent of this amount, compared to 12 percent of the average household's income spent on food (Leather 1992).

A healthy diet can be expensive. The National Children's Home compared prices of a week's 'shopping basket' of food for a family of three, at 43 locations throughout Great Britain. A basket of healthy foods including fruit, vegetables and lean meat cost an average of £33.49 and a basket of less healthy items cost £28.57, a difference of 17 percent. The difference between the cost of healthy and unhealthy foods was widest in rural areas and in Scotland. Healthier foods also tended to be less readily available in local shops, presenting another obstacle to healthy eating for low-income families unlikely to own a car (NCH 1991).

Discussion

The evidence in this chapter suggests that health education, aimed at individuals, has had limited success in altering behaviour such as teenage smoking and drug-taking. It is recognized that there are powerful influences on behaviour – such as advertising, taxation and socioeconomic circumstances – which affect the choices individuals make.

The dilemma in attempting to tackle some of these influences is that there may be a conflict between the promotion of health and 'freedoms' valued in our society. In some cases, the freedom of the individual has to be balanced against the public health, and in particular against the health of children, who may not be in a position to make their own choices. Society limits the right of the individual to enjoy drinking alcohol by making it an offence to drive over the legal limit, endangering the lives of other people.

In other cases, the conflict is between health and commercial freedom. Where a product is dangerous to health, society can choose to prohibit it completely, as with controlled drugs, limit its sale to certain outlets or to adults only, as with alcohol and tobacco, or impose other restrictions, such as on advertising.

The responsibility for balancing these conflicting interests lies with government. Ideally, legislation and policy are based on scientific evidence and reflect the values of society as a whole. The degree to which government and society are willing to restrict individual and commercial freedom to protect children's health reflects judgement on their relative value.

Still more difficult are those issues which require a balance to be struck between the interests of parents and children. Young children have no 'freedom' to choose parents who do not smoke or who do not drink heavily.

Diet is constrained by income. Parents on low incomes cannot afford fruit, green vegetables or other items which they know to be healthy. Policies on social security benefits are therefore of direct relevance to health behaviour, and reflect the relative value placed on alternative uses of public money. At the same time, commercial freedom allows the advertising of unhealthy foods, often targeted at children. Although individuals are encouraged to develop healthy lifestyles, changes in public policies will be necessary before improvements in public health can be achieved.

References

Publications other than routine data series

Action on Smoking and Health (1992) 'Tobacco advertising – the case for a ban', Brief on the proposed European Directive to ban all tobacco advertising. London, ASH.

Alberman, A. and Dennis, K. J. (1984) *Late Abortions in England and Wales: Report of a National Confidential Enquiry*. London, Royal College of Obstetricians and Gynaecologists.

Allied Dunbar National Fitness Survey (1992) London, Sports Council and Health Education Authority.

Amery, J. and Tomkins, A. (1992) 'Advertising infant formulas in hospitals', *British Medical Journal* 303: 1336.

Amos, A., Jacobson, B. and White, P. (1991) 'Cigarette advertising policy and coverage of smoking and health in British women's magazines', *Lancet* 337: 93–6.

Anderson, P. (1991) 'Alcohol as a key area', *British Medical Journal* 303: 766–9.

Beecham, L. (1992) 'EC reaches compromise on maternity benefits', *British Medical Journal* 305: 980.

Berger, N. (1990) *The School Meals Service*. Plymouth, Northcote House.

Botting, B. (1991) 'Trends in abortion', *Population Trends* 64: 19–29.

BMJ (1992) 'Headlines', *British Medical Journal* 304: 592.

Chief Medical Officer (1991) *On the State of the Public Health for the Year 1990*. London, HMSO.

Chief Medical Officer (1992) *On the State of the Public Health for the Year 1991*. London, HMSO.

Common Services Agency for the Scottish Health Service (1991) *Scottish Health Statistics 1990*. Edinburgh, CSA.

Dagg, P. (1991) 'The psychological sequelae of therapeutic abortion – denied and completed', *American Journal of Psychiatry* 148: 578–85.

Department of Education and Science (1973–90). *Annual Census of School Meals*. London, DES.

Department of Health (1988) *Present Day Practice in Infant Feeding*. Reports on health and social subjects No. 32. London, HMSO.

Department of Health (1989) *The Diets of British Schoolchildren*. London, HMSO.

Department of Health (1991) *Dietary Reference Values for Food Energy and Nutrients for the United Kingdom*. Reports on health and social subjects No. 41. London, HMSO.

Department of Health and Social Security (1974) *Present Day Practice in Infant Feeding*. Reports on health and social subjects No. 9. London, HMSO.

Department of Transport (1991) *Road Accidents Great Britain 1990: the Casualty Report*. Government Statistical Service. London, HMSO.

Emery, J. L., Scholey, S. and Taylor, E. M. (1990) 'Decline in breast feeding', *Archives of Disease in Childhood* 65: 369–72.

Ehrhardt, P. (1986) 'Iron deficiency in young Bradford children from different ethnic groups', *British Medical Journal* 292: 90–3.

Esmail, A. *et al.* (1992) 'Controlling deaths from volatile substance abuse in under 18s: the effects of legislation', *British Medical Journal* 305: 692.

Ewart, I. (1991) 'A family matter?', *Health Service Journal* 9 May: 18–20.

Fleissig, A. (1991) 'Unintended pregnancies and the use of contraception: changes from 1984 to 1989', *British Medical Journal* 302: 147.

Food Commission (1991) 'School meals best source of nutrients', *Food Magazine* 2(15).

Goddard, E. (1990) *Why Children Start Smoking*. London, HMSO.

Goddard, E. (1991) *Drinking in England and Wales in the Late 1980s*. London, HMSO.

Golding, J., Haslum, M. and Morris, A. C. (1984) What do our ten-year old children eat? *Health Visitor* 57: 178–9.

Hastings, G., Aitken, P. and MacKintosh, A. (1991) *From the billboard to the playground*. London, Cancer Research Campaign.

Health Education Authority (1992) *Tomorrow's young adults*. London, HEA.

Home Office (1991) *Fire statistics in UK 1987*. Quoted in Factsheet No. 3. London, Action on Smoking and Health.

Home Office (1991) 'Statistics of the misuse of drugs', *Statistical Bulletin* 8/91.

House of Commons Hansard (1990a) 8 February, Vol. 166, Col. 713.

House of Commons Hansard (1990b) 20 July Col. 1340.

Howie, P. W., Forsyth, J. S., Ogston, S. A., Clark, A. and Florey, C. du V. (1990) 'Protective effect of breast feeding against infection', *British Medical Journal* 300: 11–16.

Independent Scientific Committee on Smoking and Health (1988) *Fourth Report* (Froggatt Report). London, HMSO.

Lader, D. and Matheson, J. (1991) *Smoking Among Secondary Schoolchildren in 1990*. London, OPCS.

Lancet (1992) 'Young and unfit?' (Editorial), *Lancet* 230: 19–20.

Leather, S. (1992) 'Less money, less choice: poverty and diet in the UK today', in National Consumer Council, *Your Food: Whose Choice*. London, HMSO.

Matheson, J. (1991) *Participation in Sport*. General Household Survey 1987 supplement B. London, HMSO.

McKeown, T. (1976) *The Modern Rise of Population*. London, Arnold.

Ministry of Agriculture, Fisheries and Food (1990) *Household Food Consumption and Expenditure 1989*. Annual report of the National Food Survey Committee. London, HMSO.

National Children's Home (1991) *Poverty and Nutrition Survey*. London, NCH.

National Dairy Council (1982) *What Are Children Eating These Days?* London, NDC.

Northern Ireland Department of Health and Social Security (1991) *Smoking and Drinking amongst 11–15 Year Olds in Northern Ireland in 1990*. Belfast, NI, DHSS.

Northern Ireland Department of Health and Social Security (1992) *Continuous Household Survey 1/92*. Belfast, NI, DHSS.

Nutbeam, D. (1989) *Health for All Young People in Wales*. Results from the Welsh Youth Health Surveys 1986 and 1989. Cardiff, Health Promotion Authority for Wales.

Office of Population Censuses and Surveys (1992) *Infant Feeding 1990*. London, HMSO.

O'Hare, A. E. *et al.* (1984) 'Persisting vitamin D deficiency in the Asian adolescent', *Archives of Disease in Childhood*, 59: 766–70.

Price, C. and Jackson, K. (1991) 'Advertising infant formulas in hospitals', (Letter), *British Medical Journal* 303: 1058.

RCOG (1991) *Report of the RCOG Working Party on Unplanned Pregnancy*. London, Royal College of Obstetricians and Gynaecologists.

Riddoch, C., Savage, J. M., Murphy, N., Cran, G. W. and Boreham, C. (1991) 'Long term health implications of fitness and physical activity patterns', *Archives of Disease in Childhood* 66: 1426–33.

Royal College of Physicians (1992) *Smoking and the Young*. London, RCP.

Scottish Home and Health Department (SHHD) (1991) *Health Bulletin* 49/6 November.

Scottish Sports Council (1989) *School-aged Team Sport Enquiry Group Report*. Edinburgh, SSC.

Secondary Heads Association (1990) *School Sport and Physical Education*. London, SHA.

Secretary of State for Health (1991) *The Health of the Nation: a Consultative Document for Health in England*. London, HMSO.

Smith, C. (1991) 'Smoking among young people: some recent developments in Wales', *Health Education Journal* 50: 8–11.

Smith, C. and Nutbeam, D. (1992) 'Adolescent drug use in Wales', *British Journal of Addiction* 87: 227–33.

Sports Council (1990) *People in Sport: Fact Sheet*. London, Sports Council.

Wolf, J. (1992) 'Maternity law adopted', *Guardian* 20 October.

Routine data series

Office of Population Censuses and Surveys:
  OPCS AB Abortion
  OPCS FM1 Birth Statistics
  OPCS GHS General Household Survey
  OPCS Population Trends
Central Statistical Office:
  CSO Annual Abstract of Statistics (AAS)
  CSO Social Trends
Registrar General for Scotland:
  RG Scotland Annual Reports

Endpiece

Recent decades have seen improvements in many areas of child health. Mortality has continued to fall for all ages under 20 years, although markedly less for older teenagers than for younger children and infants. More low birthweight babies are now kept alive. Survival times have improved for many cancers and for certain congenital conditions such as cystic fibrosis. There have been dramatic reductions in the incidence and severity of the common childhood infectious diseases.

Not all trends are encouraging, however. Teenage deaths from suicide and solvent abuse are increasing, particularly among boys. There is some evidence to suggest an increase in the overall level of chronic illness, to which the improved survival of children with previously life-threatening conditions has contributed.

The rich and diverse data available in the UK have allowed a reasonably comprehensive review. It is important to maintain the collection of information for continued monitoring of health and the factors that influence health. However, there are many gaps in knowledge, including population-based measures of child health, detailed hospital statistics for England and Wales since 1985, and national information on the level of mental health among children. Problems of definition and measurement occur with some health states, such as 'disability', and with factors influencing health, such as 'poverty'.

We have collated evidence on possible explanations for ill-health in childhood in order to identify the major areas with potential for prevention. Several important issues have emerged.

The health of children is strongly related to their socioeconomic circumstances, children from unskilled manual households being twice as likely to die before the age of 15 as children from the professional class. The effects of adverse environments – socioeconomic, physical or cultural – tend to accumulate among children in families on low incomes and to persist into adult life. Given this well-known association, the increasing number of children living in poverty is disturbing.

Health risks from the physical environment are also widely recognized, although specific threats may be changing, especially from different sources of pollution. The knowledge on which to base an effective prevention strategy already exists for some risks, for example in accident prevention. Other hazards, such as air pollution and radiation, are less well understood and research is needed to establish their effects.

Some links between behaviour and health are well established. But behaviour is not always easy to change. It is discouraging that despite the fall in adult smoking the level of teenage smoking has been maintained, and may even be increasing among young women. It is also disappointing that the proportion of breast-fed infants has not increased in recent years.

How far does the evidence presented in this volume support the Government's choice of strategies for improving health? The Government emphasizes individual responsibility in reducing the consumption of tobacco and alcohol, preventing accidents, improving diet, increasing physical exercise and in sexual behaviour. Less emphasis is given to society's role in improving the child's environment by providing employment and housing and reducing the risk of accidents, although these are all mentioned (Secretary of State for Health 1992). The evidence presented here on the importance of socio-economic and physical circumstances for health suggests that a strategy emphasizing individual behaviour may miss important opportunities for prevention.

Reference

Secretary of State for Health (1992) *The Health of the Nation*. London, HMSO.

Note on official data sources

Information on the entire population comes from the civil registration system, which records births, marriages and deaths, and the Census. Both are the responsibility of the Registrar General and the Office of Population Censuses and Surveys (OPCS) in England and Wales and their equivalents in Scotland and Northern Ireland.

Civil – as opposed to ecclesiastical – registration began in 1837 in England and Wales and in 1855 in Scotland (Nissel 1987). The registration system today is similar, with the dual function of establishing the legal status of an individual and providing data aggregated at local and national level. Since 1975 OPCS has increased the information on infant mortality that could be derived from the separate birth and death records by linking infant deaths routinely to the social and biological information on the record of birth. More than half (58 percent) of the deaths under 20 years of age occur in infancy, but there is obvious potential for extending the system of linking to older children. The forms for recording births and deaths, showing what information is collected, are reproduced on pps 178 and 179.

The Census is the second main source of data for the entire population. Since 1801 a Census has been conducted every ten years in England and Wales, with the exception of 1941 when the war intervened. The 1991 questions included the sex and age of all members of the household, family structure, employment, qualifications and type of housing. Questions on health and ethnic group were included for the first time. It is compulsory to complete the form. The information is confidential and is used only to provide aggregate data on the population. On the same day as the Census in England and Wales, Censuses are conducted by the Registrars of Scotland and Northern Ireland. Care was taken to include the homeless in 1991, and this is important for children and teenagers.

A register of the entire population as members of the National Health Service (NHS) is maintained by OPCS. The system grew out of the population register created in 1939 to ration food and clothes and deploy labour during the war. It is kept up to date by notification of births and deaths from local registrars and notification of change of address (entailing change of general practitioner) from the local Family Health Service Authorities. On the basis of this information OPCS monitors the movement of the population within the country and forecasts local population changes. The NHS Central Register also assists medical research. The deaths of all children with cancer, for example, are notified to the cancer registries.

These data on the entire population are supplemented by national sample surveys conducted by the government. In 1970 the Government Social Survey (which had its origins in the 1939–45 war and the planning of the welfare state)

177

A.1 Registration of live birth, England and Wales

Reg Dist.		District & SD. Nos.	Entry No.	A	LIVE BIRTH	District & SD. Nos.		Entry No
Sub Dist.		Date of registration				Date of registration		

CONFIDENTIAL PARTICULARS

The particulars below, required under the Population (Statistics) Acts, will not be entered in the register. This information will be confidential and used only for the preparation of statistics by the Registrar General.

1. Where the father's name is entered in register:

   Father's date of birth   DAY   MONTH   YEAR

2. In all cases:

   Mother's date of birth   DAY   MONTH   YEAR

3. Where the child is of legitimate birth:

   (i) Date of marriage   MONTH   YEAR

   (ii) Has the mother been married more than once?   *YES   NO

   (iii) Mother's previous children (excluding birth or births now being registered) by her present husband and any former husband

   (a) Number born alive (including any who have died)

   (b) Number still-born

X   Is this birth one or more twins, triplets, etc   *YES   NO

   If YES, complete (a) and (b)

   *(a) Total number of births at this maternity

   2   3   4   5   6

   (vi)   (vii)

   Live births ——   Still-births ——

   (b) Entry No. of births   (b) Entry No. of births

FORM 309

DRAFT OF PARTICULARS OF LIVE BIRTH TO BE REGISTERED

CHILD

1. Date and place of birth

   (date) ....

2. Name and surname

   3. Sex

   L   grams

FATHER

4. Name and surname

5. Place of birth

6. Occupation

   G(a) Father

   (i)   (ii)
   (iii)   (iv)

   (va)

   H(a)*   1   2   3   4   5
   See cover for Employment Status codes

MOTHER

7. Name and surname

   G(b) Mother

8. Place of birth

9. (a) Maiden Name

   (b) Surname at marriage if different from maiden surname

   (vb)

   H(b)*   1   2   3   4   5
   See cover for Employment Status codes

10. Usual address (if different from place of child's birth)

POSTCODE

INFORMANT

11. Name and surname (if not the mother or father)

12. Qualification

13. Usual address (if different from that in 10 above)

Edit Control

Signature of registration officer by whom the above particulars were obtained

Signature of registrar registering birth on declaration

SPECIMEN

* Ring as appropriate

Office of Population Censuses and Surveys (Crown Copyright). Introduced 1 January 1986

178

A.2 Registration of death, England and Wales

Reg Dist.		District & SD Nos.		Entry No.
Sub Dist.		Date of registration		

DRAFT OF PARTICULARS OF DEATH TO BE REGISTERED

1. Date and place of death *(date)*

2. Name and surname

3. Sex

4. Maiden surname of woman who has married

5. Date and place of birth *(date)*

6. Occupation and usual address

SPECIMEN

8. Cause of death

  Ia

  b

  c

  II

Certified by

	(b) Qualification	Signature of registrar

7. (a) Name and surname of informant

  (c) Usual address

Q National Health Service medical card collected?
* YES   NO
If NO, NHS No. ....

sp/m162 5/85

DEATH

		District & SD Nos.		Entry No.
D				Date of registration

E *	6 months or over	Under 6 months	(i)	
D & SD No.		(ii)		Z

CONFIDENTIAL PARTICULARS

These particulars which are required under the Population (Statistics) Acts will not be entered in the register. This information will be confidential and used only for the preparation of statistics by the Registrar General.

Q   (iii)

At date of death the deceased was *

G(a) Deceased or †Mother

Single	1
Married 2 ⟶	
Widowed	3
Divorced	4
Not known	5

(If married insert date of birth of spouse)

Day	Month	Year

H(a)* 1 2 3 4 5   See cover for employment status codes

G(b) Husband or †Father

H(b)* 1 2 3 4 5   See cover for employment status codes

POSTCODE

J   (iv)   (v)   (vi)   (viia)   (viib)

U   1

SPECIMEN

R Last seen alive

Day	Month	Year

S * Seen or Not Seen after death
  a   b   c

T * Referred to Coroner by
  1 Doctor   2 Registrar

B SD YES NO (viii) 1 ME 2
  * Enq   3 4 5 6

N * Post
	(ix) a
Mortem	b
	c
YES	2
NO	e

M   Employment   (x)   W   1   Edit control

* Ring as appropriate   † If deceased is under 16 years of age

FORM 310

Office of Population Censuses and Surveys (Crown Copyright). Introduced 1 January 1986

merged with the General Register Office to form OPCS. From that time on, OPCS has been responsible for the regular sample surveys of the population of Great Britain on which much of the information in this book is based: the General Household Survey, the Labour Force Survey, the National Food Survey and the Family Expenditure Survey. In addition OPCS conducts surveys of special topics such as disability, smoking, alcohol and breast-feeding. Some comparable surveys are conducted in Northern Ireland, for example the Continuous Household Survey, which has been conducted since 1983.

Reference

Nissel, M. (1987) *People Count: a History of the General Register Office*. London, HMSO.

Glossary

While we have avoided specialized words and jargon as much as possible, inevitably there are terms which need some explanation. However, it would not be practical to describe here individual diseases and conditions, for which the reader is referred to a medical dictionary or textbook.

Word in *italics* denote a reference to another glossary entry.

Abortion An induced termination of pregnancy. The term 'miscarriage' is used for spontaneous loss of a pregnancy.

Admission A period in hospital including at least one overnight stay. Until 1986, 'admissions' were effectively synonymous with the official term 'discharges and deaths' except in long-stay psychiatric hospitals. The *Körner* statistics based on *episodes*, starting in 1987–8, are not directly comparable.

Becquerel A unit of radioactivity corresponding to one disintegration of an atom per second.

Birth cohort Everyone born in the same year, or other defined period of time. The three national birth cohort studies followed children born in Great Britain in one week in 1946, 1958 and 1970 and monitored their health at various ages.

Birth order The ranking of births according to age, starting with the eldest. UK statistics include *stillbirths* within marriage, but exclude both live and still births outside marriage. See also *parity*.

Birth rate The number of live births in a year divided by the total population. In the UK the birth rate per 1000 total population is about one-quarter of the birth rate per 1000 women aged 15–44, which is sometimes called the 'fertility rate'.

British Isles The *United Kingdom* and Republic of Ireland.

Carcinogenic Has been shown to cause cancer.

Casualty A person killed or injured in an accident. Road accident casualties are subdivided by the Department of Transport into killed, seriously injured and slightly injured. A 'casualty attendance' is a person attending a hospital casualty (accident and emergency) department.

Cohort A group of people with a shared characteristic, followed over a period of time. See also *birth cohort*.

Congenital anomaly A physical malformation or syndrome involving physical and/or mental problems, present at birth.

Congenital disorder A *congenital anomaly* or an inherited (genetic) condition not apparent at birth.

Consultation In general practice, any contact between a patient or his or her representative (e.g. a parent) and a doctor, including a telephone call.

Dependent child A young person aged under 16 years; or under 19 if living at home and in full-time education.

Disability   See *International Classification of Impairments, Disabilities and Handicaps.*

District   See *health district.*

Episode   In *Körner* hospital statistics, a period spent in hospital under the care of one consultant, following *admission* as an inpatient or day case. In general practice, a series of *consultations* about the same illness or complaint.

Fertility   See *birth rate* and *total fertility.*

Flow of motor vehicles   The number of vehicles passing a particular point on a road in a given period, usually 24 hours.

Gestational age   The age of a fetus or newborn baby, measured from the first day of the last menstrual period.

Great Britain (GB)   England, Scotland and Wales.

Health district   An administrative district of the NHS in England. District Health Authorities are responsible for the health of their resident population, including commissioning of hospital and community health services. The equivalent bodies in Scotland are Health Boards, while Northern Ireland is divided between four Health and Social Services Boards.

G.I   The British Isles showing English health regions

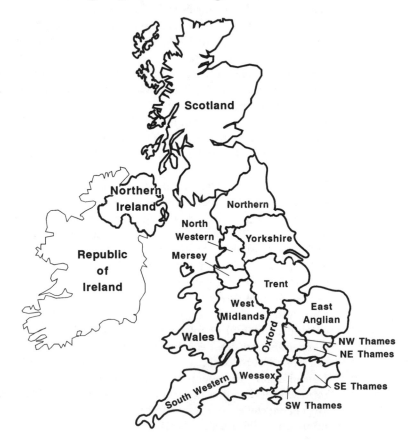

Health region Regional Health Authorities are the administrative tier of the NHS in England between *health districts* and central government. For comparison across the *United Kingdom*, Scotland, Wales and Northern Ireland are sometimes counted as equivalent to one health region each. See also *standard region*.

Household A single person or group of people who have the same address as their only or main residence and who either share one meal a day or share the living accommodation. Members of a household are not necessarily related. In the case of homeless people, the term 'household' refers to a group defined as above before they became homeless.

Immunization cover The proportion of children receiving a completed primary course of immunization by age two years (for a few immunizations the age differs).

Incidence The number of instances of a disease or other condition commencing, or the number of persons falling ill, during a given period (most often a year) in a specified population.

Infant A child under one year old; pertaining to the first year of life. Infant mortality is the number of infant deaths per 1000 live births.

International Classification of Diseases, Injuries and Causes of Death, Ninth Revision (ICD9) A system for coding causes of death, illness and use of health services for statistical purposes (WHO 1977). ICD9 is organized into 17 chapters, each containing either diseases of a particular body system (e.g. digestive system) or a particular type of condition (e.g. infectious diseases) – see Table G.1. The 'type of condition' chapters have priority over the 'body system' chapters, so that (for example) lung cancer comes under Chapter II, Neoplasms, and not Chapter VIII, Respiratory System.

Table G.1 Structure of ICD9

Chapter title		Codes	Example
I	Infectious and parasitic diseases	001–139	Measles
II	Neoplasms (cancer)	140–239	Leukaemia
III	Endocrine, nutritional and metabolic diseases	240–279	Diabetes
IV	Diseases of the blood and blood-forming organs	280–289	Anaemia
V	Mental disorder	290–319	Anorexia nervosa
VI	Diseases of the nervous system and sense organs	320–389	Cerebral palsy
VII	Diseases of the circulatory system	390–459	Rheumatic fever
VIII	Diseases of the respiratory system	460–519	Asthma
IX	Diseases of the digestive system	520–579	Inguinal hernia
X	Diseases of the genitourinary system	580–629	Cystitis
XI	Diseases of pregnancy, childbirth and puerperium	630–679	Maternal hypertension
XII	Diseases of the skin and subcutaneous tissue	680–709	Acne

Table G.1 Structure of ICD9 *continued*

Chapter title		Codes	Example
XIII	Diseases of the musculoskeletal system and connective tissue	710–739	Arthritis
XIV	Congenital anomalies	740–759	Spina bifida
XV	Conditions originating in the perinatal period	760–779	Birth trauma
XVI	Signs, symptoms and ill-defined conditions	780–799	Sudden infant death syndrome
XVII	Injury and poisoning	800–999	Fracture
E	External causes	E800–999	Motor vehicle accident
V	Factors influencing health status and contact with health services	V01–82	Immunization

Within the chapters, each condition has a three-digit code. There are a total of 1178 three-digit codes. Rare diseases do not have a unique code and so cannot be identified in routine statistics. A fourth digit (after a decimal point) gives more detail, and organizations such as the British Paediatric Association have produced lists of fifth digits to give even greater precision in their specialist areas (BPA 1979). For example:

744   Congenital anomalies of ear, face and neck
744.0   Anomalies or ear causing impairment of hearing
744.03   Anomaly of inner ear

In addition to the main codes, **E codes** (external causes) detail causes, as opposed to types, of injury and poisoning. The general heading of Injury and poisoning (E800–999) divides into E800–949 (accidents, such as motor vehicle traffic accident) and E950–999 (violence, such as suicide, homicide or physical assault). The **V codes** (supplementary classification) list reasons other than illness for contact with health services, for example receiving immunization.

In 1994 or 1995, ICD9 will be replaced in UK health statistics by the Tenth Revision, ICD10. This will have 21 chapters including the present E and V codes, in basically the same structure but identified by letters as well as numbers. For instance, Chapter II, Neoplasms, will consist of codes C00–D48. The new system of numbering allows for expansion to include new diseases (e.g. AIDS) and greater detail in some areas, so that ICD10 will contain 2033 three-digit codes (Ashley 1991).

International Classification of Impairments, Disabilities and Handicaps (ICIDH)   ICIDH is a system of classification for the consequences of disease or injury. These consequences are described at three levels: impairment, disability and handicap (WHO 1980). Impairment is any loss or abnormality of physical or mental faculties. Disability is a restriction or lack of ability to perform an activity in the manner considered normal, as the result of an impairment. Handicap is the disadvantage for a given individual, resulting from an impairment or disability, that limits or prevents the fulfilment of a normal role in society.

For example, an injury causing paralysis of the legs would result in classification to: an impairment code in the range 71–74, mechanical and motor impairments of limbs; one or more disability codes in the range 40–45, ambulation disabilities, such as code 40, walking disability; handicap scores on a number of dimensions, such as orientation, physical independence, mobility, occupation, social integration and economic self-sufficiency.

Körner The Steering Group on Health Services Information, referred to as the Körner Committee after its chair, Edith Körner; the name is also applied to the information systems set up as a result of the Steering Group's work. An important difference between pre-Körner (up to 1985) and post-Körner (1986 onwards) health service statistics is that data are now organized by financial year (starting 1 April) rather than calendar year.

Low birthweight (LBW) Low birthweight is defined as less than 2500 g (5.5 *lb*). *Very low birthweight* is less than 1500 g (3.3 *lb*).

Maternal mortality The rate per 100,000 live births of women dying as a result of complications of pregnancy, childbirth or abortion.

Maternity A pregnancy which results in one or more live or still births.

Mean The most common form of average, in which the sum of the observed values is divided by the number of observations.

Morbidity Any form of illness, disease or disability.

Mortality Number of deaths per 1000 (or another convenient multiple) of the relevant population. Except when used in a general sense, mortality is always a rate in this book.

Neonatal In the first four weeks of life. Neonatal mortality is the number of neonatal deaths per 1000 live births. The neonatal period is subdivided into early neonatal (first week) and late neonatal (the remainder).

Parity The status of a woman as regards number of previous live or still births. See also *birth order*.

Part-time Employment of 30 hours or less per week, excluding overtime.

Pedestrian casualty rate The number of pedestrian *casualties* in a year per 100,000 population at mid-year. Pedestrian mortality is pedestrian casualties killed per 100,000 population.

Perinatal From 24 weeks *gestational age* to the first week of life. Perinatal mortality is the number of perinatal deaths per 1000 *total births*.

Postneonatal After four weeks and up to the first year of life. Postneonatal mortality is the number of postneonatal deaths per 1000 live births.

Poverty The European Community recognizes a 'relative' poverty line of half the national mean household income, adjusted for household size and age of children.

Prematurity *Gestational age* of less than 37 completed weeks; failure of physiological function in a *neonate* owing to early birth.

Prevalence The number of instances of a disease or other condition in a given population at one point in time. Strictly, this is 'point prevalence', as opposed to 'period prevalence', which is the total number of persons known to have had the disease at any time during a specified period.

Proxy   A substitute or indicator used to represent something which is not measured directly. Thus, changes in hospital *admissions* might be a proxy for trends in the number of people seriously ill.

Region   Unless otherwise stated, a *health region*.

Rider   The person in control of a bicycle, motorcycle or scooter, or a ridden animal. Other occupants are counted as passengers, not riders.

Screening   The presumptive identification of unrecognized disease or defect by the application of tests, examinations or other procedures. Screening sorts out apparently well persons who probably have a disease from those who probably do not (Commission on Chronic Illness 1957). Screening may be preceded by risk identification, for example selecting pregnant women over a certain age for Down's syndrome screening. It should be followed by diagnosis, which establishes the definite presence of illness in an individual.

Sievert (Sv)   A measure of the biological effect of a given dose of radiation, which takes into account the differing capacities of different types of radiation to cause damage. In practice, one Sievert is a very large dose. Doses in the real world are most conveniently expressed in mSv (milliSieverts), thousandths of a Sievert.

Social class   A child's social class is based on the occupation of the 'head of household', conventionally the father. The social classes, defined in the Registrar General's Occupational Classification (OPCS 1980), are:

Social class		*Examples*
I	Professional	Doctor, lawyer
II	Managerial	Manager, teacher
IIIN	Skilled non-manual	Clerk, shop assistant
IIIM	Skilled manual	Miner, bricklayer
IV	Partly skilled	Bus conductor, postman
V	Unskilled	Labourer, porter
Other		Armed forces, unoccupied and inadequately described

Standardization   Two populations may have different mortality simply because they have different age structures. Age standardization is a statistical technique that permits comparison of death rates with the age structure having been taken into account. In addition to age, standardization may be used to allow for birthweight or other factors. More than one factor can be allowed for at the same time.

Standard region   A conventional division of the *United Kingdom* for statistical purposes. See also *health region*.

Stillbirth   The delivery of a dead fetus of 24 weeks *gestational age* or over (before October 1992, 28 weeks or over). The stillbirth rate is the number of stillbirths per 1000 *total births*.

G.2   The British Isles showing UK standard regions

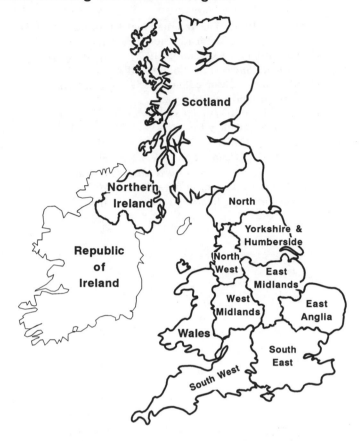

Teratogenic   Liable to cause a *congenital anomaly*.

Total births   Live births and *stillbirths* combined.

Total fertility   The number of live births a woman is likely to have if current *birth rates* continue throughout her child-bearing years.

Unemployment rate   The proportion of the labour force who are unemployed. The labour force is defined as civilians aged 16 and over who are in, or available for, employment. Some statistics are in terms of 'claimant unemployed', which means that only those claiming certain social security benefits are counted.

Unit of alcohol   To enable comparison between people consuming different types of alcoholic drink, amounts are converted to standard units containing a similar amount of pure alcohol. One unit is roughly equivalent to a half pint of beer, a single measure of spirits (1/6 gill), a glass of wine (about 4.5 fl. oz.) or a small glass of sherry or fortified wine (2 fl. oz.) (Goddard 1991).

United Kingdom (UK)   *Great Britain* and Northern Ireland.

Very low birthweight (VLBW)   Very low birthweight is defined as less than 1500 g, or 3.3 *lb*.

References

Ashley, J. (1991) 'The International Classification of Diseases: the structure and content of the Tenth Revision', *Health Trends* 22: 135–7.

British Paediatric Association (1979) *Classification of Diseases, Volumes 1 and 2 and Perinatal Supplement*. London, BPA.

Commission on Chronic Illness (1957) *Prevention of Chronic Illness*. Cambridge, MA: Harvard University Press.

Goddard, E. (1991) *Drinking in England and Wales in the Late 1980s*. London, HMSO.

Office of Population Censuses and Surveys (1980) *Classification of Occupations*. London, HMSO.

World Health Organisation (1977) *Manual of the International Statistical Classification of Diseases, Injuries and Causes of Death, Volumes 1 and 2*. Geneva, WHO.

World Health Organization (1980) *International Classification of Impairments, Disabilities and Handicaps*. Geneva, WHO.

Index